D1446578

The Eradication of Smallpox

The Eradication of Smallpox

Organizational Learning and Innovation in International Health

Jack W. Hopkins

Westview Press
BOULDER, SAN FRANCISCO, & LONDON

Westview Special Studies in Health Care and Medical Science

Copyright © 1989 by Westview Press, Inc.

Published in 1989 in the United States of America by Westview Press, Inc., 5500 Central Avenue, Boulder, Colorado 80301, and in the United Kingdom by Westview Press, Inc., 13 Brunswick Centre, London WCIN 1AF, England

Library of Congress Cataloging-in-Publication Data
Hopkins, Jack W.
    The eradication of smallpox : organizational learning and
  innovation in international health / Jack W. Hopkins.
      p.   cm.—(Westview special studies in health care and
  medical science)
    Includes bibliographies and index.
    ISBN 0-8133-7729-3
    1. Smallpox—Prevention—International cooperation.
  2. Organizational behavior. I. Title II. Series.
  [DNLM: 1. International Cooperation. 2. Smallpox—prevention &
  control. WC 588 H794e]
  RA644.S6H66   1989
  614.5′21—dc20
  DNLM/DLC
  for Library of Congress   89-16424
                                                                        CIP

Printed and bound in the United States of America

  The paper used in this publication meets the requirements of the American National
Standard for Permanence of Paper for Printed Library Materials Z39.48-1984.

10   9   8   7   6   5   4   3   2   1

For David, with love

Contents

Tables and Figures

Acknowledgments

The original stimulus for this study of the smallpox eradication campaign came from a graduate seminar on development administration at Indiana University, in which it seemed that so many cases dealt with failures. In searching for examples of successful programs, I became interested in the smallpox eradication campaign. Using some of the ideas of my colleague William J. Siffin, I pursued the research at greater length and found the story most intriguing.

Few, if any, achievements in medicine and epidemiology—or indeed in any field—surpass those of the smallpox eradication campaign. The campaign deserves to be analyzed from many perspectives; I chose to study the organization and management of the program to glean lessons that might be useful in other programs. This work owes a great deal to the work of participants in the campaign, many of whom were interviewed for this study. The Centers for Disease Control in Atlanta very kindly gave me guest researcher status and full access to its records; I am grateful to William J. Foege and his staff for their cooperation. The Smallpox Eradication Unit of the World Health Organization (WHO) in Geneva, especially Isao Arita, let me examine WHO files relating to the campaign and assisted in arranging interviews with a number of participants who were still attached to WHO. Finally, the Rockefeller Foundation provided an invaluable opportunity to work and write at the Villa Serbelloni at Bellagio, Italy. Thanks are due also to Indiana University for sabbatical time to do the basic research and to Chuo University in Tokyo for its invitation to me to serve as a visiting professor.

Especial thanks go to Katherine Arthur Hopkins, who not only encouraged me to finish the study but also typed several versions of it, and to Barbara Macy, who put the manuscript in final form.

Jack W. Hopkins

1

Smallpox as an International Health Problem

Scope of Smallpox: The Problem

By virtually any measure, smallpox ranks in the forefront of devastating diseases of human beings. When or where smallpox originated is not known. But the earliest written history refers to the scourges of the disease, which tended to affect the most densely populated areas worst— areas such as India and China where the necessary chain of transmission could be maintained. Historical accounts describe a smallpox-like disease in Europe and Africa from around the sixth and seventh centuries, and its introduction into the Americas in the sixteenth century caused the deaths of millions of the indigenous people. Much of the decline of the Aztec and Incan empires must be attributed to the decimation caused by smallpox after its spread by the Spanish conquistadores. In densely populated regions, practically the entire population was infected, and extremely high death rates resulted from the epidemics. The disease affected every continent, and practically all countries. Indeed, in many areas of the world, smallpox acted as a key factor in retarding population growth.

The spread of smallpox throughout almost the entire world by the early nineteenth century and its omnipresence in many societies, even long before recorded history, influenced civilizations and history in many ways. Tribes and kingdoms were devastated, wars were disrupted and battles lost, reigning monarchies were ended, and the deaths of countless millions of people from smallpox were so common as to be an expected part of life. Many cultures in Africa, China, and India developed deities of smallpox and prayed to them for relief from the scourge. Although early statistics on mortality are based generally only on informed estimates, it is obvious that smallpox killed enormous numbers of people throughout the world; in eighteenth century Europe some **400,000** persons died yearly from the disease and probably a third of the blindness in the continent resulted from smallpox.[1]

It is apparent, despite the dreadful impact of smallpox, that both morbidity and mortality statistics are sadly deficient in early historical accounts. Except for several clearly recorded instances, we must rely on educated estimates, projections, and extrapolations to assess the disease's impact. Yet, unfortunately, more recent statistics from many countries, especially less-developed states, are also seriously lacking. For various reasons, accurate data on the incidence of smallpox, morbidity, and mortality rates were not maintained by many countries before the intensified smallpox eradication program began in 1967. Ironically, the constant presence of smallpox in certain countries, especially in Asia and parts of Africa, led to an almost passive acceptance of the disease by both the general population and health services. The creation of deities related to smallpox reveals the deep-rooted cultural acceptance of the disease. Even health professionals and epidemiologists often adopted an attitude of resignation at the magnitude of the devastation caused by smallpox and were skeptical of the possibility of its eradication. D. A. Henderson, who directed the World Health Organization (WHO) eradication campaign for ten years, quotes a British professor's warning: "Bear in mind that Asia is the ancient home of smallpox. Eradication in Latin America or Africa is one thing; Asia is quite impossible."[2] The view expressed by A. T. Councilman further illustrates the attitudinal problem:

> Smallpox can, but probably never will be, wholly eradicated. The chief obstacle which stands in the way of its eradication is an inability to recognise facts, and to make the proper deductions from them, which seems to be associated with certain orders of mind. The facts with regard to the production of smallpox immunity by vaccinia are perfectly established. The order of mind which leads to their denial will probably never disappear from the human race.[3]

Inaccurate data reflected not only passive acceptance and resignation, but also deep-seated cultural attitudes regarding the most common victims of smallpox, especially in the densely populated endemic countries such as India, Bangladesh, and Indonesia. Commonly, smallpox was perceived as a disease of the poor, lower classes, and thus its relegation to the status of a neglected, inevitable disease. It is perhaps revealing that a 1969 article on the biopolitics of underdevelopment referred not at all to the effects of smallpox on development, even though many less damaging diseases such as tuberculosis, measles, pneumonia, enteritis, diarrhea, and others were discussed at length.[4] In fairness to the author, he does disclaim any attempt to be comprehensive. In India, there is substantial evidence that even the reporting of smallpox cases by district health officers was looked upon unkindly by health officials in upper echelons. (This problem posed serious difficulties in the early stages of the WHO eradication campaign and led to the adoption of special procedures to avoid the underreporting; these are discussed below.) Statistics from India also showed deliberate distortion; at successive levels of the health hierarchy, statistics on smallpox incidence were modified to lower the number of cases reported up the line. The result, until WHO's insistent pleading changed the situation, was thoroughly unreliable information on smallpox cases in the country. India was not alone in this. D. A. Henderson, looking back at the campaign in Bangladesh, India, Nepal and Pakistan, observed that:

> Here case detection was inadequate and reporting systems were archaic; the importance of surveillance and containment was not appreciated, and when containment was attempted, it was usually done poorly. Support for the program by health authorities was lukewarm; so many efforts to control smallpox had failed over so many years that the disease was widely considered inevitable and its elimination impossible.[5]

The public health problem simply looked different to planners in Geneva and New Delhi; this difference in perspective created major difficulties in the organization and implementation of the eradication program in India. To planners in the Ministry of Health, who saw the vast, overwhelming totality of Indian public health, perhaps smallpox was *not* the country's major health problem. To the planner in WHO, India stood out as the country that in 1973 accounted for 57.7 percent of the world's reported smallpox (in 1974, that proportion rose to 86.1 percent). The old question of relative distribution of resources continually arose; because the incidence of smallpox appeared to have declined steadily from 1967, smallpox eradication received a lower priority than, for example, malaria.[6]

The Indian planners' perspective is quite understandable, given the relative mortality rates of smallpox and other diseases. In 1973, for example, smallpox caused an estimated 15,434 deaths (0.15 percent of the total in India). But tuberculosis killed about 500,000 persons (5 percent); some 1,000,000 (10 percent) died from tetanus; diarrhea may have led to half of the childhood deaths (some 3,500,000 infants died in 1973). Estimates of malaria incidence ran to some 4,000,000 cases; leprosy, 3,720,000 cases; and tuberculosis some 5,000,000 cases.[7] Obviously smallpox, from the perspective of authorities in New Delhi, was only a small part of the overall health problem.

Speaking of the same difference of perspective in Bangladesh, Stanley Music notes:

> the enormous problems imposed by scarcity of food, clothing, materials, building materials, fuel, electricity . . . when combined with poverty of foreign exchange, high fertility, political instability and inexperience at self-government, only serve to put smallpox eradication into its real perspective. Malnutrition, gastro-intestinal diseases, and tuberculosis took many times more lives than smallpox when the SEP [Smallpox Eradication Program] began. Annually recurring epidemics of cholera held greater terror for the people than smallpox ever did.[8]

This conventional wisdom, of course, is rooted in fact. As Lane, Millar, and Neff observe,

> there has been a change in the sociologic distribution of the disease. In virtually all endemic nations smallpox is now similar to poliomyelitis and diphtheria in the United States; a disease of isolated rural villages and urban slums. Smallpox attacks those who cannot afford to be immunized, or who are not served by even minimal health services.[9]

However, the point is that a disease's prevalence just among the poorer classes is more likely to lead to neglect of the disease than if it attacked all people indiscriminately. (A parallel may be seen in the public attitude toward acquired immune deficiency syndrome—AIDS—whose saliency as a public health problem rose markedly when it became apparent that AIDS is not peculiar to homosexuals.)

The scope of the smallpox eradication problem was really unknown at the onset of the campaign. The cumulative underreporting or nonreporting of smallpox cases created worldwide an enormous gap between the number of cases reported officially and the actual incidence. Clearly, there were areas where smallpox was seriously and obviously endemic. There, as in India, Bangladesh, and Indonesia, serious data deficiencies scarcely affected the enormity of the problem. Later experience demonstrated, however, that the reporting of smallpox cases was dreadfully incomplete. Data on smallpox morbidity and mortality in many countries indicated little more than the general trend of incidence in different regions. For example, in a 1973 report, the Pan American Health Organization noted that the ratio of reported to actual cases in areas where there were no well-organized epidemiological surveillance programs might be as low as 1:40. But the magnitude of the incompleteness was surprising. D. A. Henderson observes that in 1967, 131,418 cases worldwide were reported to WHO, but there may have been that many cases in northern Nigeria alone, and for the world in 1967, a more accurate figure might fall between 10 and 15 million cases.[10]

Some diseases—smallpox was one of those—have persisted for so long in many countries that they have become, in effect, part of the fabric of the society. A severe challenge, in dealing with certain public health problems, lies in the difficulty of raising the salience of those problems out of the routine. Even a disease as dreadful as smallpox may become accepted in some cultures as an inevitable, recurrent affliction, or as a disease of the poorer classes, or as a sign of displeasure by a deity. Many of the social and economic problems of the less developed countries are rooted deeply in time, tradition, and habit. Their origins, obscured in history, are remote, and cultural and political practices for coping with such problems may become part of the problem themselves. Even in the minds of rationally calculating public health officials, diseases other than smallpox were far more destructive and, accordingly, should receive higher priority.

For many less developed countries, a complex set of social, economic, cultural, and political factors created what was, in effect, a psychological barrier[11] to confronting the full significance of a campaign to eradicate smallpox. The final successful campaign was delayed partly because the scope of the commitment intimidated the public health authorities and the governments of many countries. The enormity of the task frightened many less developed countries, many of which had come almost fatalistically to accept everpresent health crises. The World Health Organization was skeptical also. Part of the skepticism of WHO undoubtedly resulted from the failure of the malaria program. The significance of the decision itself proved to be a deterrent. The less-than-enthusiastic attitude of some countries about an eradication program perhaps reflected not incomplete understanding but rather all too complete comprehension of the difficulty of the task. As one participant observed, "perhaps we underestimated the extent to which some less developed countries understood the magnitude of the task."

Searching for a Solution

Given the enormity of the problems created by smallpox throughout much of the less-developed world, it is understandable, perhaps, why the international community acted slowly in confronting the challenge. WHO's campaign to eliminate malaria had been clearly unsuccessful. Likewise, the first attempt by WHO to attack smallpox on a global basis proved to be notably unsuccessful.

At the 1958 meeting of the World Health Assembly in Minneapolis, the Soviet Union proposed a resolution to authorize a five-year program to eradicate smallpox. For two years the primary emphasis would go to production of as much vaccine as possible, training of vaccinators among local populations, and fundraising. Then during the next three years, a mass vaccination program would be carried out to reach every unvaccinated person. The Soviet resolution was approved by the World Health Assembly meeting in Geneva in 1959, and it committed WHO to an eradication program.[12]

Given the severity of the impact of smallpox on many countries for centuries, the unwillingness of international health conferences to accept the challenge of dealing with the disease is somewhat surprising. For many years, the only diseases discussed at meetings of the International Sanitary Conferences that began in 1851 were bubonic plague, cholera, and yellow fever. None of these, despite their great impact, was as universal, destructive, and constant as smallpox. Not until 1926 did smallpox become notifiable under the International Sanitary Regulations, but even then only epidemics, not first cases, were reportable.[13] Henderson points out how "gingerly" WHO approached the smallpox problem at first. Many more years of experience from the countries of Europe and North America which had eliminated smallpox in the 1940s, and the demonstration of highly encouraging results from programs in the Philippines, Central America, and in South America by the Pan American Sanitary Bureau, were to pass before the World Health Assembly decided to take on smallpox.[14]

Several reasons may be advanced for the lack of enthusiasm among international public health officials, as well as epidemiologists. First, the sheer magnitude of the task intimidated those who contemplated eradication. None but the innocent really believed the reported statistics on smallpox cases from the less developed countries. Second, experience in these countries, as contrasted with the general success of the western industrialized countries in controlling smallpox, was in the main discouraging. In India, for example, public health workers had administered vaccinations numbering more than the total population of the country, yet smallpox persisted strongly. Third, there were still doubts about the technology for mass vaccination. The failure of earlier eradication efforts was due in part to poor vaccine quality and unsatisfactory vaccination implements—for example, the painful rotary lancet was still used in many areas. Finally, experience was lacking in the kind of large-scale, international cooperation in public health that would be necessary for a worldwide attack on smallpox. And, of course, the first WHO eradication program, starting in 1959, was a failure. All these factors combined to make WHO, organizationally, less than eager to undertake another eradication program.

Tracing the genesis of any public health program to a precise point is always difficult; the smallpox eradication program is no exception. The long postponement by the World Health Assembly of a decision to undertake a worldwide campaign to eradicate smallpox reveals the importance of what might be termed "appropriate timing" in public administration. For many reasons, the 1959 eradication programs failed, and that failure contributed to the problem of "appropriate timing" for approval of the 1966 campaign. Timing, indeed, may have been a factor as critical as appropriate technology in the second (successful) smallpox eradication campaign. One participant/observer described the 1959 campaign as a "rhetorical exercise." The campaign operated on very limited resources, these depending on voluntary contributions from member states, and the more developed countries offered insufficient support. Much of the emphasis in the 1959 program went to vaccine production rather than operational efforts, although there were certain exceptions such as Peru, Ivory Coast, and Senegal.

However, despite the priority given to vaccine production, sufficient quantities of potent vaccine of consistently high quality were not produced. Several countries started mass vaccination campaigns, but except in China, these programs failed. A general shortage of vehicles, equipment, manpower, and funds plagued the campaign. There was no special budget in WHO for the 1959 smallpox program and no focal organizational unit or effective management control. These problems, combined with delays in organizing national programs, failure to produce understanding and popular support, and poor coordination between countries (resulting in reintroduction of smallpox across borders), doomed the 1959 program to failure. A further obstacle existed, because to some developing countries, smallpox was "not the most important public health problem."[15]

In many countries, skepticism about the prospects of a successful eradication program was well supported. In West Pakistan, for example, vaccination against smallpox began in 1875. In recent decades, before 1970, 14 million vaccinations per year were performed in a population of some 46 million. "Although presumably enough to break the chain of infection, no corresponding decline in disease incidence has been evident."[16]

It is important to note, in order to appreciate the critical role of precise problem definition, that the Soviet proposal of 1958 contained the outline of a campaign strategy based upon mass vaccination: ". . . the problem of smallpox eradication throughout the world is to a large extent reduced to the eradication of the principal endemic foci of this disease *by means of the vaccination of the whole populations.*" (italics added). An economic rationale also clearly underlay the proposal:

It should also be noted that our proposals are strongly supported by the economic considerations. . . . It is quite clear that the cost of uncoordinated smallpox vaccination carried out in various countries over a number of years exceeds the sums that would be required for a coordinated campaign against smallpox in endemic areas.[17]

In many respects, the 1966 eradication campaign was "a case of the right place at the right time." Fortunately, when the U.S. Agency for International Development (AID) wanted the Communicable Disease Center (CDC) to assume responsibility for the measles campaign in West Africa, CDC's price was "smallpox too." AID had wanted to omit Nigeria because of its size, but CDC insisted that Nigeria be included.[18] Some observations about the measles campaign are highly critical of the AID role:

> The measles program was anything but a success and my feeling, shared by other colleagues, was that AID hindered more than helped international health. Nevertheless, the fiasco led the CDC to capitalize on the mistakes, and press for a smallpox program. In a series of steps, AID reluctantly shifted its emphasis from measles to smallpox.[19]

It is really not clear what the politics of the agreement were. Some believe that AID was "bludgeoned" by CDC to accept a vertical program in West Africa, but at least one major participant thinks it was almost the reverse.[20] Whatever the facts of the West Africa AID-CDC agreement, it is clear that the successful campaign in that region was a dramatically important factor in building momentum and optimism to undertake the intimidating problem of Asia. The measles/smallpox campaign began in 1966. In January 1967, with support from AID, CDC, and WHO, twenty countries of West and Central Africa began a coordinated campaign of smallpox eradication. Some 40 percent of the population of the area were vaccinated by July 1968, a total of some 47 million persons.[21] Early victories in West Africa, especially after use of the surveillance-containment strategy, "encouraged and electrified the whole campaign." Many people in India were doubtful even then, however.[22]

Without doubt, WHO's second smallpox eradication program was one of the most outstanding successes in the history of public health. Probably no other accomplishment in the ancient struggle against disease exceeds the importance of the final eradication of smallpox. Given the failure of the 1959 smallpox eradication program of WHO, why was the second eradication campaign, commencing in 1967, successful? This study focuses principally upon that question.

The accomplishments of the smallpox eradication campaign have been chronicled widely from technical and journalistic perspectives.[23] Those aspects of the campaign are well known. However, little systematic attention has been given to the organizational and management implications of the smallpox campaign.[24] The successful program to eradicate smallpox exemplifies not only superior technical and epidemiological achievements but also organizational learning and innovation of the first order. These aspects—organizational learning and adaptive innovation— have vitally important implications for future efforts in international health administration. It is the hypothesis of this study that *success of well-conceived technological and scientific applications and programs, in both short-run and long-range perspectives, may depend as much or more on administrative, management, and organizational aspects as on the technology and science involved.* The smallpox eradication program was a "victory for sound epidemiology" and also "an enormous amount of slogging" by non-medical workers.[25] Study of the organization and management of the campaign offers lessons which have direct and indirect applications for other programs of communicable disease control and public health administration at both the national and international levels. It is beyond the scope of this study to even attempt a detailed analysis of the smallpox eradication campaign in individual countries. (That task has been undertaken by WHO in a series of analyses of country campaigns and by other studies of separate campaigns. In 1988, as this study neared completion, WHO's encyclopedic work on the campaign was published.)[26]

The purpose here, rather, is to review the overall, worldwide smallpox eradication program with the objective of deriving general conclusions which may be expressed in terms of instructive lessons for future health programs. This analytical review required the use of examples from several individualized country programs of the overall eradication effort, mining of the extensive official records of WHO, and interviews of participants in the eradication campaign, principally personnel of WHO in Geneva and the Centers for Disease Control in Atlanta.

Before undertaking that review and analysis, however, it is essential that the disease itself—smallpox—be understood. An assessment of the success of the eradication campaign and any prediction of applicability to other diseases and other health programs must take into account the special characteristics of smallpox. This task is undertaken in the next chapter.

Notes

1. WHO. *The Global Eradication of Smallpox.* Final report of the Global Commission for the Certification of Smallpox Eradication (Geneva: WHO, 1980), p. 16.

2. Donald A. Henderson, "Smallpox—Epitaph for a Killer?" 154 *National Geographic* (December 1978), 804.

3. W. T. Councilman. *Selected Essays on Syphilis and Smallpox. Translation and Reprints from Various Sources.* Edited by A. E. Russell (London: New Sydenham Society, 1906), p. 189. Cited by Stanley I. Music in *Smallpox Eradication in Bangladesh: Reflections of an Epidemiologist.* Dissertation submitted to the London School of Hygiene and Tropical Medicine, 1976.

4. Robert B. Stauffer, "The Biopolitics of Underdevelopment," 2 *Comparative Political Studies* (October 1969), 361–387.

5. D. A. Henderson, "The Eradication of Smallpox," 235 *Scientific American* (October 1976), 31.

6. Lawrence B. Brilliant. *The Management of Smallpox Eradication in India* (Ann Arbor: The University of Michigan Press, 1985), pp. 29–31.

7. Statistics from Brilliant. *The Management of Smallpox Eradication in India,* p. 31.

8. Stanley I. Music. *Smallpox Eradication in Bangladesh: Reflections of an Epidemiologist.* Dissertation submitted to the London School of Hygiene and Tropical Medicine, University of London, 1 June 1976, pp. 6–7.

9. J. Michael Lane, J. Donald Millar, and John M. Neff, "Smallpox and Smallpox Vaccination Policy," 22 *Annual Review of Medicine* (1971), 265.

10. Donald A. Henderson, "The Eradication of Smallpox," 235 *Scientific American,* (October 1976), 30.

11. Dr. Donald R. Hopkins, Assistant Director, Centers for Disease Control, suggested this concept to me.

12. Shurkin observes that WHO and its Director-General, Marcelino Candau, were not enthusiastic, having been unsuccessful in the earlier malaria campaign. Joel Shurkin, *The Invisible Fire: The Story of Mankind's Victory Over the Ancient Scourge of Smallpox* (New York: G. P. Putnam's Sons, 1979). I could not confirm or disprove his allegation during my interviews, although it was clear that many in WHO did not then believe eradication was possible.

13. Norman Howard-Jones, "Thousand-Year Scourge," *World Health* (February/March 1975), 5.

14. Donald A. Henderson, "The Eradication of Smallpox," 235 *Scientific American* (October 1976), 28.

15. K. Rasha, "Global Eradication of Smallpox." Ninth International Conference for Microbiology, Moscow, July 1966. WHO Doc. SE/66.2.

16. M. B. Khawaja, "Surveillance Activities of the Smallpox Eradication Programme in West Pakistan." WHO Doc. WHO/SE/71.30, p. 195. (This evidence was actually used in 1971 to support the surveillance/containment strategy, but it also illustrates the previous point.)

17. 87 WHO *Official Records* (1958), pp. 508–512.

18. Interview, Stanley Foster (CDC), 7 May 1981.

19. Lawrence K. Altman, "The Doctor's World: The Eradication of Smallpox." *The New York Times,* 16 October 1979, p. C3.

20. Interview, J. Michael Lane (CDC), 15 May 1981.

21. William H. Foege, J. Donald Millar, and J. Michael Lane, "Selective Epidemiologic Control in Smallpox Eradication," 94 *American Journal of Epidemiology* (October 1971), 311–312.

22. Interview, Donald Hopkins (CDC), 6 May 1981.

23. The following are examples of works that treat the campaign from the epidemiological perspective: W. H. Foege, *et al.*, "Current Status of Global Smallpox Eradication," 93 *American Journal of Epidemiology* (April 1971), 223–233; "Selective Epidemiologic Control in Smallpox Eradication," 94 *American Journal of Epidemiology* (October 1971), 311–315; Donald A. Henderson, "Epidemiology in the Global Eradication of Smallpox," 1 *International Journal of Epidemiology* (Spring 1972), 25–30; "Surveillance of Smallpox," 5 *International Journal of Epidemiology* (March 1976), 19–28; C. Kaplan, "Symposium on Smallpox Eradication," 69 *Transactions of the Royal Society of Tropical Medicine and Hygiene* (1975), 293–298; and *Smallpox Eradication* 393 WHO Technical Report Series (1968), pp. 5–52. Other accounts, more reportorial and descriptive, include Donald A. Henderson, "The Eradication of Smallpox," 235 *Scientific American* (October 1976), 25–33; John H. Douglas, "Death of a Disease," 10 *Science News* (February 1975), 74–75; and *World Health* (February/March 1975 and May 1980), entire issues devoted to the smallpox campaign.

24. An exception is the study by Lawrence B. Brilliant, *The Management of Smallpox Eradication in India* (Ann Arbor: The University of Michigan Press, 1985). This work was extremely valuable in providing specific examples of some of my major points. The monumental *Smallpox and Its Eradication*, by F. Fenner, D. A. Henderson, I. Arita, Z. Jezek, and I. D. Ladnyi (Geneva: WHO, 1988), is the definitive account of the eradication campaign.

25. Interview, Donald Millar (CDC), 15 May 1981.

26. See, for example, *Smallpox Eradication in Nepal*, WHO/SE/78.107; *Smallpox Eradication in Thailand*, WHO/SE/78.113; *Smallpox Eradication in Ethiopia*, WHO/SE/79.144; *Smallpox Eradication in Somalia*, WHO/SE/79.145, and other country reports of WHO.

2

Smallpox: Characteristics, Epidemiology, and Control

Characteristics

Several characteristics of smallpox qualified the disease as a unique target for worldwide eradication.[1] Some of these characteristics contributed importantly to the success of the smallpox eradication program. The smallpox virus is acquired when tiny droplets of aerosolized virus are inhaled from a sick patient. The inhaled virus infects the epithelium (cellular tissue) of the bronchiolar and upper respiratory tract, multiplies in epithelial cells, and then localizes in lymph nodes, tonsils, and adenoids. A primary viremia follows; this ends when the virus is cleared from the bloodstream by the cells of the reticuloendothelial system. In these cells, the smallpox virus again multiplies extensively and is released in massive amounts in a secondary viremia. The result is fever, muscular pain (myalgia), and malaise, and infection of skin and internal organs, leading to the characteristic eruption of skin and mucous membrane. Approximately 12 days elapse between the initial infection after inhalation of the virus and the secondary viremia, and after about 14 days the clinically apparent rash begins its onset. These are two strains of variola virus. One, *variola minor,* causes fatality of less than one percent. The other, *variola major,* has a fatality rate ranging from 20 to 40 percent among unvaccinated persons.[2]

A. R. Rao has classified the principal types of smallpox according to the nature and evolution of the lesions; this classification was useful in prognosis and field investigations.[3] In the *ordinary type,* which is the most frequent, making up some 85 percent of cases, the febrile, preeruptive illness lasts from two to four days, and as the eruption develops, the patient's temperature usually drops. On the third or fourth day of illness, skin lesions appear as papules; fluid begins to collect in them, usually within 24–48 hours. The lesions are sharply raised and begin to dry and scab from the eighth to the tenth day after eruption. Generally, there is a parallel between the severity of the clinical picture and the extent of the rash.

The *modified* clinical type, accounting for some 5–7 percent of cases, occurs in vaccinated persons. The pre-eruptive illness is usually less severe than in the ordinary type; secondary fever may not occur, and skin lesions are often few. They tend to evolve more quickly, are more superficial, and may not show the typical uniformity. Modified type cases are never fatal.

The *flat* type, also accounting for about 5–7 percent of cases, with severe pre-eruptive illness and fever persisting throughout the eruptive phase, is frequently fatal. Lesions mature slowly and the vesicles tend to be flat, projecting little from the skin. In patients who survive, the lesions resolve without pustulation.

The *haemorrhagic* clinical type, accounting for less than one percent of cases, is almost invariably fatal. The pre-eruptive illness is accompanied by fever, intense headache and backache, restlessness, a facial flush or pallor, extreme prostration, and toxicity. The fever is likely to continue without remission throughout the illness. Haemorrhagic manifestations may appear on the second or third day and death often occurs suddenly between the fifth and seventh days of illness, when only a few lesions are present. In patients who survive for 8–10 days, the haemorrhages appear in the early eruptive stage.

The clinical appearance of patients infected with smallpox virus aids substantially in identification. The ordinary type of smallpox, making up some 85 percent of cases, is readily recognized. Diagnosis of the flat and modified forms is also relatively easy. But even experienced physicians may miss cases of the haemorrhagic type. In terms of the clinical course of smallpox, the incubation period typically runs from 10–12 days after exposure until the onset of illness. The pre-eruptive phase, accompanied by fever, headache, muscular aching, prostration, and often nausea and vomiting, then starts abruptly. Two or three days later, the rash begins, followed over a period of one week by lesions that progress to form vesicles and then pustules. Scabs form over the next week and fall off over a period of one to two weeks. During the acute phase, most cases are easily recognized. For several weeks or months after recovery, characteristic depigmented areas remain, and are helpful in discovering recent cases of smallpox. Former victims of smallpox carry facial pockmarks.[4]

Fortunately, most cases of smallpox were typical—of the ordinary clinical type—so that experienced health workers could readily recognize them. Chickenpox most closely resembled smallpox, so that sometimes even experienced observers confused the two, especially in mild or modified cases of smallpox. For this reason, during the latter phases of the eradication campaign, the Smallpox Eradication Unit in WHO placed much emphasis on definitive laboratory diagnosis of specimens obtained from outbreaks of chickenpox. Some other diseases, such as measles, syphilitic rash, scabies, monkeypox, as well as infected insect bites and drug eruptions, sometimes caused difficulties in diagnosis. But for the great majority of cases, diagnosis was relatively straightforward and the field teams could proceed directly to vaccination without delay. This was a critical advantage in the overall eradication campaign.[5]

Epidemiology of Smallpox

Thus, the characteristics of smallpox facilitated its identification and eradication. Writing on the epidemiology of smallpox, Lane, Millar, and Neff observe:

> Smallpox is uniquely susceptible to total world-wide eradication. There is no host or reservoir of the disease other than man. There are no subclinical carriers. Only close, generally identifiable, contacts of cases acquire the disease. Patients with sufficient infection to transmit the disease are overtly ill; even those with attenuation of the disease from prior vaccination get marked prodromal symptoms although their rash may be minimal.[6]

Many people attribute the success of the smallpox eradication program to the fact that smallpox was "the right disease at the right time." Essentially what this means is that smallpox is an easily recognized disease; it is a disease greatly feared by the public; it is a disease for which prevention is simple and effective; and the results can be seen easily or made obvious by information devices.[7] One participant has observed that:

> The smallpox program was fortunate in that it could deal with humans only, avoiding problems of mosquito resistance [as in malaria and yellow fever control programs] and the formidable difficulties of environmental control [as in polio and tetanus].[8]

Residual immunity from vaccinations may attenuate smallpox and reduce risk of death. But mild cases may go unrecognized and help spread the disease because they are not isolated. They are not efficient vectors because of the small number of lesions.[9]

Careful analysis of the patterns of smallpox incidence revealed unexpected epidemiological characteristics. These, in turn, helped stimulate changed strategies for dealing with the problem. For example, it was assumed originally that reported cases from a country or region would be dispersed widely through that area. However, usually the disease was quite localized. In 1967, in a district in Pakistan of 1,000,000 people, 1,040 cases were found; but only 10 percent of the 1,700 villages were infected. In India that year, in a very endemic region, only 4.3 percent of 2,331 towns were infected *throughout* the year, and no more than 20 towns (1 percent) at any one time. These findings further indicated the value of surveillance-containment measures for coping with smallpox outbreaks.[10]

It was also discovered that transmission of the aerosolized smallpox virus at considerable distance was unlikely; similarly, few outbreaks occurred as a result of contact with blankets, clothes, and scabs of former patients. Almost all cases occurred as a result of very close contact with patients, generally only in the same household. The belief that smallpox would occur in explosive outbreaks with hundreds of cases in a single incubation period was not substantiated by field observations. The disease came to be understood as "chains of transmission that required renewal, through infection of new persons, every two or three weeks." Thus smallpox could be stopped with well-directed containment measures focused on specific outbreaks, in order to interrupt the chain of transmission.[11]

Smallpox is clearly less infectious than measles or influenza. The disease generally spreads to close contacts of infected cases: family members, members of the same household, health care personnel, and others who come into close contact. Epidemiologically, this pattern enhances the susceptibility of smallpox to control by careful investigation of cases, identification and tracing of contacts, and then vaccination of persons even potentially exposed. In effect, a ring of immunized persons is created around each case. (This strategy is discussed at length under the chapter on organizational learning.)

The prevalent belief that smallpox was one of the more contagious infectious diseases[12] was not substantiated by field observations. Transmission is rarely to more than two or three persons and typically occurs within the infected household. It also typically involves only a small percentage of villages at a given time. There is an interval between generation of cases of two weeks or more.[13]

Differences in patterns of spread were discovered between *variola major* and *variola minor*. The patient was usually immobilized by *variola major*, so that secondary cases occurred typically in the immediate vicinity of the primary care. On the other hand, patients with *variola minor*, a much milder disease as a rule, remained ambulatory and were likely to spread the infection far more widely. This complicated the tracing of transmission chains and made containment and eradication more difficult because of the lack of concern that many communities felt for the milder form of smallpox.[14]

TABLE 2.1 Transmission Patterns of Smallpox

Locale of Infection	OUTBREAKS				
	U.K. 1961-62	Sweden 1963	Kuwait 1967	Abakaliki Nigeria 1967	Bawku Ghana 1967
Imported	5	1	1	1	(?) 2
Household (or compound)	17	13	1	30	58
Hospital & other medicine	39	13	32	0	0
Market	0	0	0	1	3
Other & Unexplained	6	0	8	0	5
Totals	67	27	42	32	68

Source: D. A. Henderson, "Smallpox Surveillance in the Strategy of Global Eradication." See endnote 15.

Studies done by Henderson show that transmission most commonly occurs as a result of close contact as in a household, hospitals, or school. Casual contact results relatively infrequently in transmission. Table 2.1 shows these patterns.[15]

Successful vaccination reduces the risk of smallpox to virtually nil for from three years (for *variola major*) to seven years (for *variola minor*). Twenty years after vaccination, little protection remains. In the incubation period, primary vaccination affords some protection if given three or four days after exposure. For partially immune persons, revaccination during the incubation period may abort the disease as late as seven to eight days after exposure.[16]

Early Prevention

Ironically, there was nothing new about the means for prevention of smallpox. The basic scientific and medical knowledge about the causes and effects of smallpox, and the technology for immunization against the disease by means of vaccination, had been available since the pioneering experiments of Edward Jenner in 1796. It was common knowledge, well before Jenner's work, that persons who had already had cowpox could not be infected with smallpox. Country milkmaids, who frequently caught cowpox, did not contact smallpox. Some deliberate inoculation with cowpox had been employed years before Jenner's experiments.

Antedating such inoculation by centuries was the practice of variolation (deliberate inoculation) with smallpox virus, used in Africa, India, and China before its introduction into Europe and North America in 1721. Variolation consists of scratching pustular material from an infected person's skin into a healthy person's skin. The objective of variolation was not to prevent smallpox, but to induce immunity by a less severe infection than would likely be experienced if the disease were contacted by the natural inhalation of the smallpox virus into the respiratory system. Thus it was intended to protect some people against the worst effects of smallpox. Variolation, of course, frequently resulted in death for the variolated person. The practice gradually disappeared as the smallpox eradication campaign reduced the number of cases. The practice of variolation ended in Ethiopia, where its last known use occurred in 1976, with the last smallpox outbreaks. (In a bit of novel adaptation by the smallpox eradication teams, some traditional variolators were converted to vaccinators using freeze-dried vaccine.)

The significant contribution of Dr. Jenner in 1796 was not the inoculation of people with cowpox, but his proving that such persons were immune to smallpox by later inoculating them with smallpox. Despite some problems, including occasional unintended infections of smallpox, Jenner's vaccination technique was recognized rapidly as a safe means to protect against smallpox. Vaccine was shipped to other physicians in Europe and America and Jenner's treatise, *An Inquiry into the Causes and Effects of Variola Vaccine, a Disease, Discovered in some of the Western Counties of England, Particularly Gloustershire, and Known by the Name of Cow Pox,* was translated into several languages. In 1803, King Charles IV of Spain, in a unique technique, transferred vaccine to overseas Spanish colonies by means of vaccinating a chain of children arm-to-arm in succession during the voyage. Throughout Europe, governments began to require vaccination of citizens and the incidence of smallpox steadily dropped. The problems sometimes caused by arm-to-arm passage of cowpox virus—such as the spread of syphilis and hepatitis—were solved by Dr. Negir of Naples, who passed vaccine material from cow to cow and then inoculated people from the infected cattle. Eventually dried vaccines were developed in France and Germany, and in the 1950s, a method for the production of freeze-dried vaccine was developed, solving the problem of using vaccine in tropical areas.[17]

Thus, the scientific, technical, and medical base, in effect, was essentially in place when the smallpox eradication campaign began in 1966—discovery or invention of a new technology was not the problem. Although

TABLE 2.2 Countries Reporting Smallpox & No. of Endemic Countries

Year	Countries Reporting Smallpox	No. of Endemic Countries
mid- 1940s	80	N.A.
1966	43	28
1970	23	14
1971	16	11
Dec. 1971	8	8

Source: Department of HEW, Vaccination Against Smallpox in the United States: A Reevaluation of the Risks and Benefits (Feb. 1972).

technological advances continued as the eradication program developed—improvements such as the jet injector, high-quality freeze-dried vaccines, and the bifurcated needle—*some of the most critical variables in the campaign proved to be those of problem definition, organization, and management.* We turn to those considerations in Chapter 3.

Previous Control Programs

Because of various national control programs throughout the world, the geographical area in which smallpox was endemic shrunk steadily. (Smallpox is endemic in a country when there is indigenous transmission not directly associated with importation.) The decrease in the number of endemic countries (see Table 2.2) was accomplished by a sharp decline in the total number of smallpox cases in the world.[18] Table 2.3 indicates the reported smallpox cases by continent from 1963 to 1971. The dramatic decline in countries reporting smallpox cases is shown graphically by Figure 2.1. (As pointed out above, however, the data or reported cases from Africa and Asia should not be considered definitive before 1968.) A similar, dramatic decline in the number of smallpox cases in the United States occurred from 1920 to 1950, as shown by Table 2.4.

At the beginning of the world smallpox eradication program in 1967, many separate national and international eradication or control projects were already underway. All the endemic African countries were conducting more or less intensive programs. WHO-assisted projects were underway in the Ivory Coast, Upper Volta, Liberia, Mali, Nigeria, Sierra Leone,

Table 2.3 Reported Smallpox Cases by Continent, 1963-1971

Continent	1963	1964	1965	1966	1967	1968	1969	1970	1971
Africa									
North	5	-	-	-	-	-	-	-	-
West & Central	6,687	3,565	6,257	7,599	10,818	5,408	476	-	-
South & East	10,249	9,058	10,699	6,897	4,460	5,549	3,119	3,090	26,659
South America	7,385	3,713	3,632	3,665	4,537	4,375	7,410	1,795	19
Asia	108,405	58,906	91,558	76,184	111,340	64,766	43,032	25,841	24,102
Europe	129	-	1	72	5	2	-	22	-
TOTAL	132,860	75,242	112,147	94,417	131,160	80,100	54,037	30,812	50,780

Source: WHO. Weekly Epidemiological Record 1972, 47, #6.

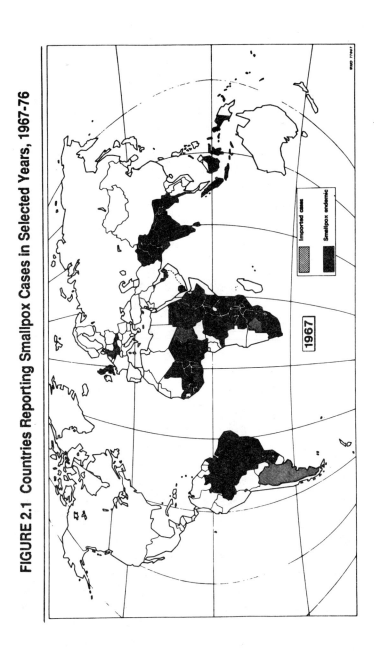

FIGURE 2.1 Countries Reporting Smallpox Cases in Selected Years, 1967-76

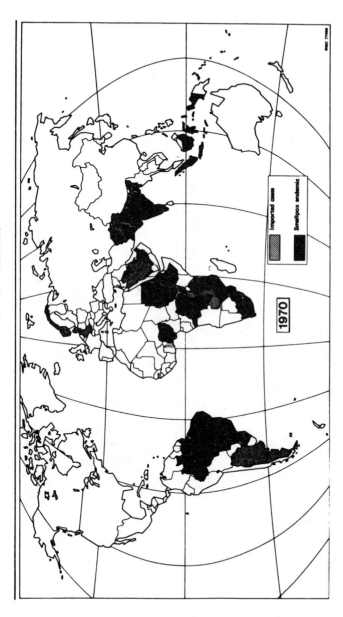

COUNTRIES REPORTING SMALLPOX CASES IN 1970

1970

Imported cases

Smallpox endemic

22

FIGURE 2.1 (Continued)

COUNTRIES REPORTING SMALLPOX CASES IN 1973

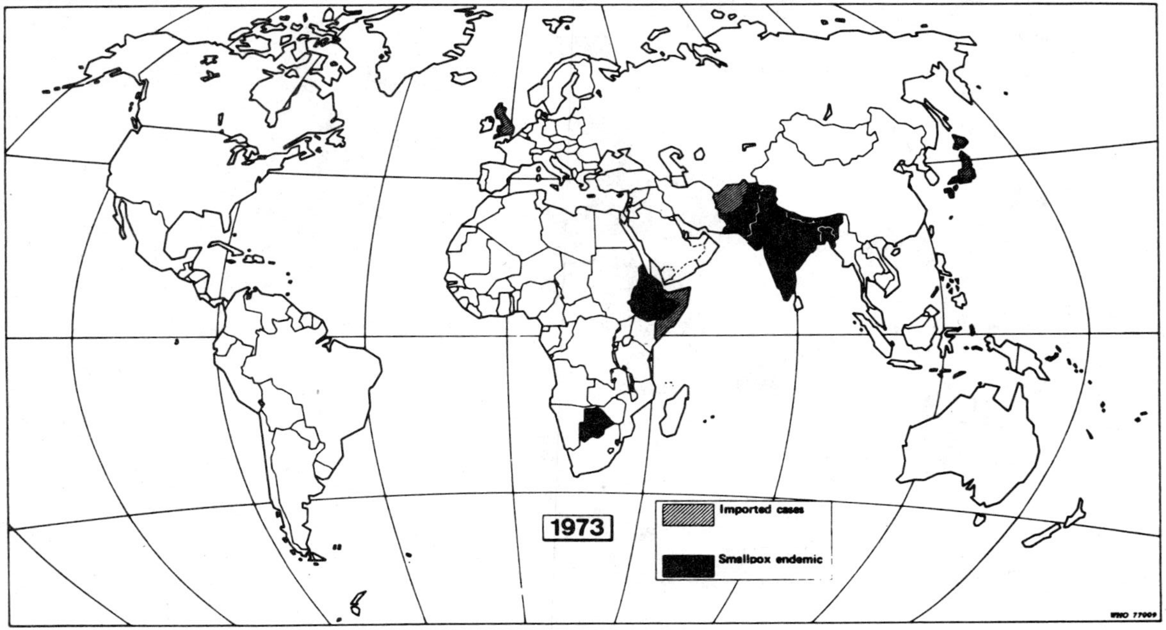

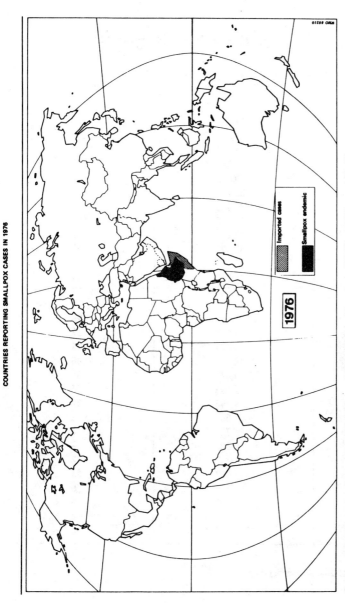

COUNTRIES REPORTING SMALLPOX CASES IN 1976

1976

Imported cases

Smallpox endemic

Source: WHO. The Global Eradication of Smallpox. (Geneva: WHO, 1980), pp. 40-41.

TABLE 2.4 Smallpox Cases in the United States—1920-1950

Year	Number of Cases	Number of Deaths
1920	102,128	498
1921	102,787	620
1922	33,378	607
1923	30,907	126
1924	56,591	871
1925	39,572	707
1926	33,732	376
1927	37,600	138
1928	39,396	129
1929	42,282	137
1930	48,907	165
1931	30,233	93
1932	11,224	38
1933	6,491	39
1934	5,371	24
1935	7,957	25
1936	7,834	35
1937	11,673	34
1938	14,939	48
1939	9,877	41
1940	2,795	14
1941	1,396	12
1942	865	2
1943	765	8
1944	397	9
1945	346	12
1946	337	25
1947	176	5
1948	57	5
1949	49	2
1950	39	

Source: Centers for Disease Control, 1981.

TABLE 2.5 Reported Smallpox Cases and Deaths in Brazil, 1956-1969

Year	Population[a]	No. of Cases	Incidence Rate[b]	No. of Deaths	Case-Fatality Rate (%)
1956	26,646,000	4,718	17.7	55	1.2
1957	27,313,000	2,661	9.7	36	1.4
1958	30,694,000	2,190	7.1	72	3.3
1959	29,467,000	4,840	16.4	93	1.9
1960	45,371,000	6,561	14.5	173	2.6
1961	67,952,000	8,526	12.5	143	1.7
1962	73,087,000	9,763	13.4	165	1.7
1963	76,409,000	6,467	8.5	163	2.5
1964	76,211,000	3,168	4.2	69	2.2
1965	78,587,000	3,417	4.3	45	1.3
1966	77,492,000	3,623	4.7	29	0.8
1967	86,580,000	4,514	5.2	70	1.6
1968	89,376,000	4,372	4.9	38	0.9
1969	92,282,000	7,407	8.0	37	0.5

[a] Estimated population of areas covered by notification system
[b] Per 100,000 estimated population

Source: Eurico Suzart de Carvalho Filho, Leo Morris, Arlindo Lavigne de Lemos, Juan Ponce de Leon, Alberto Escobar, and Oswaldo José da Silva, "Smallpox Eradication in Brazil, 1967-69," 43 Bulletin of the World Health Organization (1970), p. 798.

Togo, Sudan, and Zambia. In the Americas, a regional eradication program started in 1950 and was successful in many countries, but smallpox was re-established in Colombia and Peru. Argentina started a national campaign in 1961 and was planning another in 1966. Colombia and Peru reinstituted mass vaccination programs. Brazil in 1966 was the worst Latin American case; its eradication program started in 1962 and was continuing still in 1966. (See Table 2.5.)

In Asia, most of the endemic countries started mass vaccination campaigns between 1960 and 1962. Of these, Ceylon, Malaysia, the Republic of Vietnam, Singapore, and Thailand rid themselves of smallpox. The six remaining endemic countries (Afghanistan, Burma, India, Indonesia, Nepal, and Pakistan) were in various stages of developing or continuing national vaccination programs underway in 1966. Despite WHO assistance, Afghanistan had not yet developed a systematic program. Burma's campaign was operating successfully and the mass campaign was to be completed in 1966. India started its campaign in 1962, planning to complete it in 1966. Indonesia, although it had drawn up an eradication plan, had not implemented it by 1966. The WHO-assisted program in Nepal, started in 1961, was limited mainly to the Kathmandu Valley. East Pakistan completed a mass vaccination program in 1964, but a large number of cases were still being reported in 1965. A similar situation held in West Pakistan in spite of intensification of the vaccination program in 1965.[19] Figure 2.1 shows the declining number of countries reporting smallpox from 1967 to 1976 and Table 2.6 portrays the sequence of eradication in forty-three countries as the campaign progressed.

In most of the industrialized, western countries, smallpox vaccination had become compulsory by the end of the nineteenth century. As the disease declined dramatically throughout Europe, to the point where the rare cases that occurred were due to importation, compulsory vaccination was dropped by a number of countries. For example, England ended compulsory routine smallpox vaccination in the 1950s. Ninety percent of the British population, as of 1972, had never been vaccinated or had not been vaccinated in the previous ten years. The British experience demonstrated that routine childhood vaccination was not necessary to prevent the spread of smallpox if adequate containment measures were taken whenever the disease was imported. (Only ten imported cases were reported between 1960 and 1972.) England's experience with control was very similar to that of other European countries which had even higher immunity levels in the population.

In spite of the then prevalent belief in the United States that smallpox would spread rapidly and uncontrollably if cases were imported, the European experience in the 20 years after 1950 did not support the belief. Nevertheless, for many years, the dominant health policy in the United States required compulsory routine childhood vaccination. The overall costs associated with the protection of the United States against smallpox were very substantial. Axnick and Lane in their 1972 study document U.S. protection costs in 1968 to amount to approximately $154 million. As Tables 2.7 and 2.8 indicate, the costs were largely due to direct costs of vaccination, including time lost from work, physicians' fees, and costs for treatment of vaccination complications. These costs are summarized in Figure 2.2. (The Axnick and Lane analysis actually was produced to emphasize the relatively low cost of the worldwide eradication campaign as well as to provide a rationale for continued U.S. support for such international programs. The WHO smallpox eradication campaign, by comparison, appeared to be a bargain.)

In a similar analysis, Sencer and Axnick examined costs and benefits connected with the delivery of immunization services (principally for smallpox and measles) and reached approximately the same conclusions.

TABLE 2.6 The Sequence of Eradication in 43 Countries of Africa, South America, and Asia

Area	Country	1967	1968	1969	1970	1971	1972	1973	1974	1975	1976	1977	1978
WEST AFRICA	Senegal	1	·	·	·	·	·	·	·	·	·	·	·
	Ivory Coast	2	·	·	·	·	·	·	·	·	·	·	·
	Liberia	6	5	·	·	·	·	·	·	·	·	·	·
	Ghana	114	24	·	·	·	·	·	·	·	·	·	·
	Upper Volta	195	100	·	·	·	·	·	·	·	·	·	·
	Mali	292	131	1	·	·	·	·	·	·	·	·	·
	Guinea	1,530	334	12	·	·	·	·	·	·	·	·	·
	Niger	1,187	679	28	·	·	·	·	·	·	·	·	·
	Benin	815	367	58	·	·	·	·	·	·	·	·	·
	Sierra Leone	1,697	1,143	80	·	·	·	·	·	·	·	·	·
	Togo	332	784	83	·	·	·	·	·	·	·	·	·
	Nigeria	4,753	1,832	182	79	·	·	·	·	·	·	·	·
SOUTH AMERICA	Fr. Guiana	·	1	·	·	·	·	·	·	·	·	·	·
	Uruguay	·	2	3	·	·	·	·	·	·	·	·	·
	Argentina	30	·	·	24	·	·	·	·	·	·	·	·
	Brazil	4,514	4,372	7,407	1,771	19	·	·	·	·	·	·	·
CENTRAL AFRICA	Chad	86	1	·	·	·	·	·	·	·	·	·	·
	Uni. Rep. Cameroon	59	87	15	·	·	·	·	·	·	·	·	·
	Burundi	74	301	108	197	·	·	·	·	·	·	·	·
	Rwanda	·	·	107	253	·	·	·	·	·	·	·	·
	Zaire	1,479	3,800	2,072	716	63	·	·	·	·	·	·	·
	Indonesia	13,478	17,350	17,972	10,081	2,100	34	·	·	·	·	·	·
SOUTH & EAST AFRICA	Lesotho	1	·	·	·	·	·	·	·	·	·	·	·
	Zambia	47	33	·	2	·	·	·	·	·	·	·	·
	Swaziland	25	20	24	·	·	·	·	·	·	·	·	·
	Mozambique	104	145	11	·	·	·	·	·	·	·	·	·
	S. Rhodesia	26	12	25	6	·	·	·	·	·	·	·	·
	Unit. Rep. Tanzania	1,629	455	117	32	·	·	·	·	·	·	·	·
	Malawi	38	61	65	39	9	·	·	·	·	·	·	·
	S. Africa	43	81	246	121	10	·	·	·	·	·	·	·
	Sudan	9	106	130	1,051	1,141	827	·	·	·	·	·	·
	Uganda	365	55	9	2	19	16	·	·	·	·	·	·
	Botswana	1	·	·	·	36	1,059	27	·	·	·	·	·
INDIAN SUB-CONTINENT	Burma	2	181	68	·	·	·	·	·	·	·	·	·
	Afghanistan	334	739	250	1,044	736	236	25	·	·	·	·	·
	Bhutan	6	3	·	·	·	·	6	3	·	·	·	·
	Pakistan	6,084	1,836	3,520	3,192	5,808	7,053	9,258	7,859	·	·	·	·
	Nepal	110	249	163	76	215	399	277	1,549	95	·	·	·
	India	84,902	35,179	19,281	12,773	16,190	27,407	88,114	188,003	1,436	·	·	·
	Bangladesh	6,648	9,039	1,925	1,473	-	10,754	32,711	16,485	13,798	·	·	·
HORN OF AFRICA	Djibouti	·	·	·	·	26	93	14	13	·	·	·	·
	Ethiopia	466	426	197	722	26,329	16,999	5,414	4,439	3,935	915	·	·
	Kenya	153	87	14	·	46	·	·	4	·	·	5	·
	Somalia	·	·	·	·	·	5	7	11	14	39	3,229	·

Source: WHO. The Global Eradication of Smallpox. (Geneva: WHO, 1980), p.86.

TABLE 2.7 Estimated Economic Costs Associated with Protection of the United States
Against Smallpox—1968

	Amount
A. Costs of Smallpox Vaccination and Complications of Vaccination	$135,656,000
B. 1. Costs of Traffic Clearance and International Surveillance	6,462,000
2. Cost of Time Lost by Maritime Industry in Waiting for Clearance	8,000,000
C. 1. Cost of United States Support to World Health Organization of Smallpox Programme	699,000
2. Cost of Assistance to Smallpox Eradication Efforts in 19 Countries in West Africa	2,959,000
Total Economic Cost	$153,776,000

Source: WHO Doc. WHO/SE/72.45

An important by-product of the analysis is its contribution toward answering the critical policy question about the most rational distribution of resources between domestic protection and international disease eradication. Clearly, a close and direct international relation exists between international disease eradication and domestic protection policy.

A similar situation existed in the United Kingdom and Sweden. Sencer and Axnick analyzed the cost of smallpox importations into these two areas. In 1961 and 1962, importations of smallpox into England and Wales with a secondary spread of 62 cases cost approximately $3.6 million. Importation into Sweden in 1963, with a resultant 27 cases, cost some $750,000, including costs of isolation and vaccination reactions. The important point is that these importation costs would have been incurred regardless of the normal costs of routine vaccinations, and only worldwide eradication would eliminate much costs.[20]

Previous U.S. programs to control or prevent smallpox were based on four features:

1. routine vaccination of the population
2. vaccination of travelers

TABLE 2.8 Estimated Economic Costs Associated with Smallpox Vaccination for the Civilian Population, United States—1968

		Amount
Direct Costs		$93,460,000
Physician Services		
Office Care		
Vaccination Administration	$91,454,000	
Vaccine	1,346,000	
Complications of Vaccination	280,000	
Hospital Care		
Complications of Vaccination	25,000	
Hospital Services		
Complications of Vaccination	132,000	
Institutional Care for Mentally Retarded*	45,000	
Vaccinia Immune Globulin, Drugs	78,000	
Surveillance of Complications of Vaccination	100,000	
Indirect Costs		$42,196,000
Earnings lost due to time off work for vaccinations and complications of vaccinations	41,705,000	
Earnings lost due to premature death as a result of complications of vaccination*	378,000	
Earnings lost due to permanent disability as a result of complications of vaccination*	113,000	
Total Economic Cost		$135,656,000

*Future years discounted at 6%

Source: WHO Doc. WHO/SE/72.45

FIGURE 2.2 Economic Cost Associated with Protection of the United States
Against Smallpox, 1968

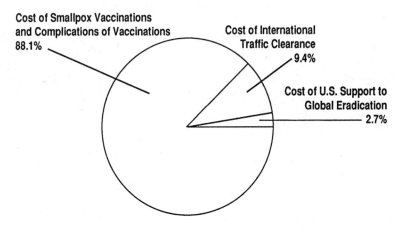

Cost of Smallpox Vaccinations
and Complications of Vaccinations   Cost of International
88.1%   Traffic Clearance
                                         9.4%

                                         Cost of U.S. Support to
                                         Global Eradication
                                         2.7%

Source: D. J. Sencer and N. W. Axnick, "Cost Benefit Analysis," International Symposium on Vaccination
Against Communicable Diseases, Monaco, 1973, p.39.

3. inspection of vaccination certificates of returning travelers and
immigrants
4. investigation of suspect cases, with rapid isolation and control
(This, of course, was an early form of the surveillance-containment
strategy used so successfully in the global campaign.)

In the United States, some 15 million vaccinations were performed
each year, of which six million were primary. The costs (including vaccine
production, vaccination fees, time lost for vaccination, maintenance of
the foreign quarantine system, research, and medical costs of vaccination
complications) were estimated to be $147 million yearly.[21] Lane and his
colleagues point out that as of 1970, the U.S. immunity level was relatively
low. Seven percent of the population was vaccinated each year; 11 percent
had never been vaccinated; less than 20 percent had been vaccinated
within three years. Therefore, 11 percent had *no* immunity to smallpox
and 50 percent had insufficient immunity to prevent the disease. Their
conclusion was that "elimination of sources of smallpox in other countries
will do more to protect the United States than will maintenance of this
uncertain immunity in the U.S. population."[22]

Reviewing the risks of introduction of smallpox, Lane and his colleagues
noted that recent U.S. experience resulted in fewer than the average
number of cases and deaths than in recent European experience. An
introduction into Texas in 1949 resulted in eight cases and one death;

in New York City in 1947, there were twelve cases and two deaths. Both areas were poorly immunized. "Pre-existing levels of immunity did not prevent importation, and did little to control spread." Their conclusion was that "importations into the United States could probably be contained by outbreak investigation and selective vaccination of contacts."[23]

As a result of recommendations of the Public Health Service Advisory Committee on Immunization Practices, which assessed the risk of smallpox in the United States to be so small as to no longer justify the practice of routine smallpox vaccination, the Public Health Service in 1972 recommended that smallpox vaccination as a routine, nonselective procedure be terminated in the United States.[24]

The costs and benefits of eradication of smallpox, when projected on a worldwide basis, showed a dramatic ratio of costs to benefits. In tracing the development of support for the eventually successful campaign which began in 1967, one can see the gradual growth of determination to proceed. One of the threads that formed the fabric of resolve consisted of a rudimentary type of cost-benefit analysis, never very complete. The original Soviet proposal of 1958, as noted above, was founded partly on economic considerations. Others noted the relative advantages to the developed countries in a successful eradication campaign. K. Raska observed that vaccination and revaccination costs in smallpox-free countries were so high that

> the additional cost of 3 years' routine vaccination would be sufficient to cover a ten-year eradication programme which would lead to the eradication of smallpox from the globe . . . the increased expenditure on the smallpox eradication program in developed countries would pay itself back within three years after the achievement of eradication.[25]

However, it would be misleading to suggest that the ultimate adoption of the smallpox eradication program depended to any substantial degree on rational cost-benefit analysis. Many epidemiologists and public health officials, of course, were generally aware of the worldwide costs, both direct and indirect, of protective measures against smallpox. But the single most frequently cited cost-benefit analysis of the eradication campaign was essentially post facto. Further, that analysis dealt primarily with U.S. domestic costs, and came at a time when the second WHO campaign was fully engaged.[26]

There were no detailed benefit-cost analyses conducted prior to the global eradication program. In 1966, as one participant observed, "thinking was small." There were no WHO "management types" who carried out such economic analyses before the 1966 proposal to proceed was adopted. WHO, *after* the global eradication campaign had succeeded,

estimated that worldwide costs of routine vaccination programs, quarantine services, control of international travelers, and medical care of
complications caused by vaccination amounted to about $1 billion per
year.[27]

In summary, the record reveals little rational cost-benefit analysis in
WHO prior to the eradication campaign. Indeed, as one interviewee
suggested, there was much discussion in WHO about the need for such
analyses, but almost nothing was done—possibly, in part, because these
calculations might have shown disparate benefits to the developed countries. (The Axnick and Lane study, as a matter of fact, showed exactly
that; the U. S. share of the costs of the global eradication campaign was
less than 3 percent of the U.S. expenditures for smallpox protection in
1968.)[28]

The Sencer and Axnick cost-benefit analysis provided additional support,
again post facto, for the WHO eradication campaign and for U.S. financial
and personnel contributions to the program:

> The savings in delivery of routine vaccinations and the medical services
> associated with complications between 1971 and 1972 are valued at $63.5
> million. The results clearly indicate that the public policy decision to
> discontinue routine vaccination of the general population released substantial
> resources for other uses.
>
> . . . In summary, this analysis indicates the costliness of an internationally
> important and emotionally fearful infectious disease in a country where
> the disease has not occurred since 1949. It also suggests that the magnitude
> of global benefits of the forthcoming worldwide eradication of smallpox
> is substantial, and the importance of the WHO smallpox eradication program
> as a part of our national protection strategy in order to realize the full
> benefits of the policy change.[29]

The WHO decisional process, although not based in this instance on
its own economic analysis, not surprisingly appears to have been motivated,
in large part, by calculations of the self-interest of major participants,
at least the Soviet Union and the United States. Humanitarianism as
well was clearly a strong factor in the ultimate decision. The record of
the World Health Assembly reveals how cooperation in health programs
continued in the face of acrimony over various political issues. At the
24th World Health Assembly, for example, the Soviet Union offered to
increase its contributions of smallpox vaccine, and in the next breath
condemned U.S. aggression in southeast Asia and Israeli aggression in
the Middle East.[30]

The WHO Director-General noted in his report to the 19th World
Health Assembly that costs of vaccination, even in the non-endemic

TABLE 2.9 General Cost Estimates (U.S. $million)

Year	1967	1968	1969	1970	1971	1972	1973	1974	1975	1976	Total
Total Estimated Cost	22.0	31.0	35.0	31.0	25.0	14.0	13.0	7.0	1.5	0.5	180.0
Share of International Assistance	6.7	7.7	8.9	7.7	5.9	4.1	3.8	2.5	0.8	0.5	48.5

Source: WHO Official Records, 151. A19/P&B/2, 28 March 1966, p.121.

countries, were high. For example, Czechoslovakia estimated its annual expenditures on maintenance vaccination to be over $1 million; the United States expended $20 million annually; and the United Kingdom in a normal year spent $650,000. (A smallpox outbreak in 1961 and 1962 raised expenditures in the U.K. to approximately $3.8 million.)[31]

In the same report, in which the broad outlines and timetable for the worldwide eradication campaign were spelled out, the Director-General estimated that the total cost of the ten-year program would be $180 million. Program cost estimates are shown in Table 2.9.

These cost projections were based on theoretical assumptions of the cost in African countries, revisions of existing program costs in Southeast Asian countries, and past experience in Latin America and parts of Africa. As a base cost, the estimates used $.10 per vaccination for a projected 1.790 billion vaccinations during the ten years. (See Table 2.10.) It was assumed that the entire population of endemic countries would be vaccinated during the campaign.[32]

Final actual costs of the smallpox eradication program from 1967 to 1979, including estimated national expenditures, were approximately $313 million. Thus, *the total cost of worldwide eradication was only twice the annual cost of previous smallpox protection for the United States alone.* Table 2.11 summarizes expenditures and contributions for the campaign. International assistance from many countries, as indicated by Table 2.12, made up a major portion of the eradication program budget. Total contributions received or pledged are shown in Table 2.13.

Numerous studies have been carried out since certification of eradication, showing costs and benefits of the program. For example, Brilliant's analysis of the Indian eradication campaign indicates that "India recoups

TABLE 2.10 Estimated Population to be Vaccinated with International Assistance
(Population in Millions)

WHO Region	Total Population			Estimated Population to be Vaccinated with International Assistance										
	1966	1970	1974	1967	1968	1969	1970	1971	1972	1973	1974	1975	1976	Total
Africa	170	190	220	20	60	80	60	50	50	50	30	10	-	410
The Americas	140	160	180	40	60	60	30	30	30	30	-	-	-	280
South-East Asia	650	710	780	130	150	170	170	150	40	40	30	-	-	880
Eastern Mediterranean	140	150	170	30	40	40	50	20	20	10	10	-	-	220
TOTALS	1,100	1,210	1,350	220	310	350	310	250	140	130	70	10	-	1,790

Source: WHO Doc. A19/P&B/2, p.120

TABLE 2.11 Expenditure on Smallpox Eradication, 1967-1979 (US$)[a]

	Estimated Expenditure 1967-1979	% of Total
International Expenditure		
WHO Regular Budget	33,565,248	11
WHO Voluntary Fund for Health Promotion	37,643,037	13
Other Organs of United Nations System	2,492,328	1
Bilateral Assistance	24,269,124	8
Total	97,969,737	33
National Expenditure in the Endemic Countries[a]	200,000,000	67

[a] Based on analysis of financial data from Bangladesh, Ethiopia, India and Indonesia and less complete data from other countries which had endemic smallpox in 1967.

Source: F. Fenner, D. A. Henderson, I. Arita, Z. Jezek, and I.D. Ladnyi. Smallpox and Its Eradication (Geneva: WHO, 1988), p. 1366.

TABLE 2.12 International Assistance to Smallpox Eradication; Yearly Contributions 1967-1979 (US$ millions)

	WHO Budget[**]	USA[*]	USSR[*]	Sweden	Other Countries[*]	Total
1967	2.73	2.56	1.83	-	0.06	7.18
1968	3.04	2.85	1.91	-	0.11	7.91
1969	3.11	2.62	1.91	-	0.07	7.71
1970	3.17	2.78	2.16	-	0.06	8.17
1971	3.25	2.81	2.22	0.10	0.41	8.79
1972	3.51	2.93	1.03	-	0.78	8.25
1973	3.26	0.79	1.03	-	0.87	5.95
1974	3.51	1.04	0.46	3.24	1.04	9.29
1975	4.34	1.09	0.37	6.28	4.49	16.57
1976	3.68	3.42	0.45	2.91	3.00	13.46
1977	2.77	1.85	-	1.57	2.34	8.53
1978	1.22	1.50	-	1.59	2.97	7.28
1979	.34	-	0.65	-	0.42	1.41
	37.93	26.24	14.02	15.69	16.62	110.50
1980	-	-	0.65	-	-	0.65
1981	-	-	0.65	-	-	0.65
	37.93	26.24	15.32	15.69	16.62	111.80[***]

[*] Includes bilateral assistance
[**] Includes headquarters, estimated at $400,000 per year 1967-1977
[***] Rounding error accounts for difference between this figure and $112 million total in next table.

Source: WHO. The Global Eradication of Smallpox (Geneva: WHO, 1980), p. 106.

TABLE 2.13 Contributions for Smallpox Eradication in Cash or in Kind to the
WHO Voluntary Fund for Health Promotion, Special Account for Smallpox Eradication,
and from Sources of Bilateral Support, 1967-1979 (US$)

Contributor	Total	Voluntary Fund for Health Promotion, Special Account for Smallpox Eradication		Bilateral Support (Cash and Kind)
		Cash	Kind	
Australia	33, 625	33, 625	-	0
Austria	75,500	5,000	-	70,500
Argentina	13,275	-	13,275	0
Belgium	378,800	-	378,800	0
Brazil	128,925	-	128,925	0
Cameroon	707	707	-	0
Canada	2,505,061	1,306,779	1,156,282	42,000
Colombia	3,002	-	3,002	0
Czechoslovakia	41,118	-	41,118	0
Denmark	1,083,062	1,083,062	-	0
Finland	110,623	19,663	90,960	0
German Democratic Republic	26, 417	-	26, 417	0
Germany, Federal Republic of	503,767	127,004	-	376,763
Ghana	3,272	3,273	-	0
Greece	23,000	23,000	-	0
Guinea	18,529	-	18,529	0
Hungary	33,500	-	33,500	0
India	503,691	-	207,291	296,400
Iran	874,000	500,000	374,000	0
Japan	634,198	268,400	223,598	142,200
Jordan	140	-	140	0
Kenya	168,000	-	168,000	0
Kuwait	12,992	12,992	-	0
Luxembourg	6,541	6,541	-	0
Monaco	2,419	-	2, 419	0
Netherlands	2,803,133	2, 613,393	177,870	11,870
New Zealand	10,500	-	10,500	0
Nigeria	16,036	16,036	-	0
Norway	998,530	998,530	-	0
Peru	3,000	-	3,000	0
Philippines	5,000	-	5,000	0
Poland	3,500	-	3,500	0
Saudi Arabia	200,000	200,000	-	0
Sweden	15,689,584	15,408,504	281,080	0
Switzerland	372,169	118,659	219,910	33,600
Thailand	3,565	-	3, 565	0
Uganda	12,077	12,077	-	0
Union of Soviet Socialist Republics	8,805,610	-	3,531,913	5,273,697
United Kingdom	1,020,924	1,010,924	-	10,000
United States of America	24,974,003	6,339,900	1,258,408	17,375,695
Yugoslavia	26,000	-	26,000	0
Zaire	2,500	2,500	-	0
Council of Arab Ministers' Fund for Health Development	20,350	-	20,350	0
Japan Shipbuilding Industry Foundation	1,769,344	1,769,344	-	0
OXFAM	103,104	3,104	-	100,000
Tata Iron & Steel Co. Ltd. (India)	536,399	-	-	536,399
Other	52,238	26,806	25,432	0
Subtotal	64,611,731	31,909,823	8,432,784	24,269,124

TABLE 2.13 (Continued) Contributions for Smallpox Eradication in Cash or in Kind to the WHO Voluntary Fund for Health Promotion, Special Account for Smallpox Eradication, and from Sources of Bilateral Support, 1967-1979 (US$)

Contributor	Total	Voluntary Fund for Health Promotion, Special Account for Smallpox Eradication		Bilateral Support (Cash and Kind)
		Cash	Kind	
UNDP (United Nations (Development Programme)	299,344	-	-	299,344
UNDRO (Office of the United Nations Disaster Relief Coordinator)	470,849	-	-	470,849
UNEO (United Nations Emergency Operation	750,000	-	-	750,000
UNICEF (United Nations Children's Fund	427,878	-	-	427,878
UNROD (United Nations Relief Operation, Dacca)	415,500	-	-	415,500
Subtotal	2,363,571	-	-	2,363,571
Total	66,975,302	31,909,823	8,432,784	26,632,695

Source: *Smallpox and Its Eradication*. (Geneva: WHO, 1988), p. 464.

its total investment in smallpox eradication by a tenfold margin" *each year*. Likewise, the United States recoups its total contribution to the global eradication campaign ($21 million) *every 26 days*. Similar analysis indicates that the world recoups its total expenditures for eradication (some $312 million) *every four months*. By virtually any measure, the investment in the smallpox eradication campaign was one of the best investments ever made—by both more-developed and less-developed countries.

Notes

1. This description of the characteristics and epidemiology of smallpox is drawn principally from J. Michael Lane, J. Donald Millar, and John M. Neff, "Smallpox and Smallpox Vaccination Policy," 22 *Annual Review of Medicine* (1971), 257–272, and *WHO Expert Committee on Smallpox Eradication*. Second Report. WHO Technical Report Series No. 493. (Geneva: WHO, 1972).

2. I. Arita, "Virological evidence for the success of the smallpox eradication programme," 279 *Nature* (24 May 1979), 295.

3. Cited in A. M. Ramsay and R. T. D. Edmond, *Infectious Diseases* (London: Heinemann, 1967), as cited by WHO Expert Committee on Smallpox Eradication, pp. 20–22.

4. WHO. *The Global Eradication of Smallpox*. Final Report of the Global Commission for the Certification of Smallpox Eradication. (Geneva: WHO, 1980), pp. 19–20.

5. *Ibid.*, p. 20.

6. Lane, Millar, and Neff, "Smallpox and Smallpox Vaccination Policy," 264.

7. N. A. Ward, "Use of Techniques learnt in smallpox eradication as applied to the prevention of blindness." Consultative meeting on Prevention of Visual Impairment and Blindness, New Delhi, 24–26 March 1976. WHO SEA/Opthal. Meet./16, 24 March 1976.

8. Brilliant. *The Management of Smallpox Eradication in India,* p. 148.

9. Lane, Millar, and Neff, "Smallpox and Smallpox Vaccination Policy," 251–272, and D. A. Henderson, "Surveillance—The Key to Smallpox Eradication." WHO/SE/68.2.

10. WHO. *The Global Eradication of Smallpox,* (Geneva: WHO, 1980), p. 32.

11. *Ibid.*

12. As in F. H. Top, Sr. *Communicable and Infectious Diseases,* 6th edition (St. Louis: C. V. Mosby Co., 1968), pp. 465–473, and O. Felsenfeld. *The Epidemiology of Tropical Diseases* (Springfield, Ill.: Charles C. Thomas, 1966), pp. 336–343, as cited in William H. Foege, J. Donald Millar, and J. Michael Lane, "Selected Epidemiologic Control in Smallpox Eradication," 94 *American Journal of Epidemiology* (October 1971), 311–315.

13. William H. Foege, *et al.,* "Selected Epidemiologic Control . . .", 311.

14. WHO. *The Global Eradication of Smallpox.* (Geneva: WHO, 1980), p. 23.

15. Source: D. A. Henderson, "Smallpox Surveillance in the Strategy of Global Eradication." Inter-Regional Seminar on Cholera and Smallpox, Malaysia and Singapore, 11–18 November 1972.

16. J. Michael Lane, *et al.,* "Smallpox and Smallpox Vaccination Policy," 255. In the early twentieth century, the risks of vaccination complications were considered insignificant compared to the risk of smallpox. Lane and his colleagues review more recent data on complications. The most common central nervous system complication is post vaccinial encephalitis. Dermal complications include accidental infection, erythematous urticargial eruptions, generalized vaccinia, eczema vaccinatum, and vaccinia necrosum. Other complications include fetal vaccinia, rare inflammatory conditions such as myocarditis, arthritis, and perhaps sudden death in infants. But data are insufficient to indicate that vaccination is unacceptably risky. Lane, *et al.,* 257–264.

17. WHO. *The Global Eradication of Smallpox,* pp. 17–18.

18. Source: Tabulated from data in U.S. Department of Health, Education, and Welfare. *Vaccination Against Smallpox in the United States: A Reevaluation of the Risks and Benefits.* (February 1972).

19. WHO Doc. A19/P&B/2, 28 March 1966, pp. 111–114.

20. D. J. Sencer and N. W. Axnick, "Cost Benefit Analysis." International Symposium on Vaccination against Communicable Diseases, Monaco, 1973. Symp. Series immunobiol. Standard, vol. 22, 37–46.

21. J. Michael Lane, *et al.,* "Smallpox and Smallpox Vaccination Policy," 251.

22. *Ibid.,* 256.

23. *Ibid.,* 265–266.

24. U.S. Department of Health, Education, and Welfare. *Vaccination Against Smallpox in the United States: A Reevaluation of the Risks and Benefits.* 1972.

25. K. Rasha, "Global Eradication of Smallpox," International Congress for Microbiology, Moscow, July 1966. WHO Doc. SE/66.2, p. 6.

26. Norman W. Axnick and J. Michael Lane, "Costs Associated with the Protection of the U.S. Against Smallpox." WHO Doc. WHO/SE/72.45.

27. WHO. *The Global Eradication of Smallpox* (Geneva: WHO, 1980), p. 64.

28. Axnick and Lane, "Costs Associated with the Protection of the U.S. Against Smallpox," 1.

29. Sencer and Axnick, "Cost Benefit Analysis," 40–41.

30. WHO *Official Records,* 194. 24th World Health Assembly, 4–20 May 1971, p. 122.

31. WHO *Official Records,* 151. A19/P&B/2, 28 March 1966, p. 106. The source of WHO data is not known; obviously there is a large difference from U.S. reports, especially the cost-benefit analyses cited above. The difference probably stems from different calculation of indirect costs.

32. WHO *Official Records,* 151. A19/P&B/2, 28 March 1966, p. 121.

3

Organization and Management

There are some virtues in not being fully able to foresee all the problems which the future holds.
—Letter, D. A. Henderson (WHO) to Stanley O. Foster (CDC)
24 August 1970

It has been emphasized that the flexible mode of management followed by the small WHO headquarters staff of the smallpox eradication campaign contributed vitally to the organization's ability to learn and innovate. The overall record and the campaign's performance appears to support that conclusion. At the same time, however, the campaign created administrative and philosophical fallout that even today is felt strongly in WHO, CDC, and other organizations concerned with international health. It is the purpose in this section to examine the organization and management of the program and some of the questions that were raised by the global smallpox eradication campaign.

Interviews of many of the leading actors in the campaign organization itself, the World Health Organization, and the Centers for Disease Control revealed surprisingly tender sensitivities about the overall operation. These concerns ranged from reactions to strong personalities to interagency conflict to country roles in the global campaign to broad questions of vertical, special purpose organizations versus integrated health care systems in international health. It is impossible in the scope of this work to deal comprehensively with all these issues. Instead, I will attempt to focus on the flexible mode of management of the campaign and discuss its effectiveness in relation to some of the other problems.

Management of Information

Although the management mode was flexible and open (one participant described it as "ad hockery" all the way),[1] the campaign nevertheless relied upon careful planning and setting of goals, continual assessment, and rapid response to field requests for assistance and advice. D. A. Henderson, who directed the ten-year campaign from WHO headquarters in Geneva, observed that such field requests "were accorded absolute priority requiring immediate response."[2]

Summaries of the campaign's progress were published regularly in the WHO *Weekly Epidemiological Record.* One participant observed, "The *Weekly Epidemiological Record (WER)* hadn't changed in all its existence." Henderson argued that information must get back to endemic countries— feedback was essential. But there was "tremendous resistance" to adding smallpox data to the *WER.* Eventually the Smallpox Eradication Unit was able to add such data to a reprint of the *WER* and send this version to its own mailing list. Another troublesome problem was persuading countries to accept the data on smallpox incidence which was generated by the smallpox campaign as country data. It was very difficult to sell the idea that reporting more cases was good.[3] Henderson observes, in regard to the *WER* modification: "Although this represented the essential last link in the surveillance process, it was difficult to persuade WHO senior officials."[4]

Special papers were published on results of research, approaches, and operational methods. The reporting-surveillance system concentrated on *trends in the incidence of smallpox,* not the number of vaccinations or how completely areas were covered. At time, publication of such trends caused severe criticism of the campaign. For example, in India, in 1973, the intensive surveillance-reporting system indicated an increase in the number of recorded cases, and the Indian press interpreted the increase to mean that the campaign had failed. In reality, the data signalled success, because surveillance was working effectively to locate cases and the tight containment strategy was slowing the spread of smallpox.

Improvements of reporting systems and data management were crucially important to the campaign's success. We have referred above to the very large disparity between officially reported cases and the actual incidence of smallpox.[5] Basu estimated that in India less then one-tenth of the cases was reported to central health officials in 1967.[6]

> For many reasons, . . . smallpox data which were available to and published by WHO through much of the 1960's, bear only a vague resemblance to the smallpox situation as it actually was. The quality of data reflected the interests and responsibilities of those concerned. . . . Underlying problems in the system at WHO, however, were essentially no different than the problem in each of the countries.[7]

After 1967, governments were asked by the WHO project staff to submit reports of smallpox cases (and no cases) promptly each week.

Smallpox unit staff scrutinized each report and queried strange or unusual reports. Conflicting reports were reconciled. Deliberate suppression of case reports apparently occurred in only a few countries, and these were identified through the unofficial smallpox information network (reports from returning travelers, health professionals, etc.). Most governments reversed their policies quickly when approached frankly. (Records and data were computerized in 1969.)

Underreporting continued to be a major management problem during much of the campaign. Either through neglect or design, case reporting was notoriously deficient in many countries, and the problem occupied much of the attention of headquarters staff. In India and Bangladesh, for example, there were strong pressures on district and local health authorities *not* to report cases of smallpox and, not infrequently, data underwent change as the statistics filtered upward in the reporting system. The Smallpox Eradication Unit in WHO found it difficult to persuade health ministry officials that the urgency of smallpox eradication demanded special reporting channels. The problem had existed in India long before the intensified WHO campaign began. Gelfand's observations are revealing:

> Cases are often hidden to escape detection: the patient and his family often accept the disease as a visitation of the goddess Shitala Mata . . . and many wish to avoid compulsory hospitalization; the family and neighbors often wish to avoid the investigation and vaccination that may follow; the sanitary inspector may prefer not to know about a small episode that might cause a considerable amount of vaccination work; and the local medical offices may to report an outbreak that reflects upon the vaccination status of community that is his responsibility.[8]

As a means to improve the timeliness and accuracy of field reports, the campaign found it necessary to provide incentives. These incentives held out positive inducements to performance and also facilitated accurate rather than "good" or "expected" reporting and performance. In India, for example, serious underreporting of smallpox cases had resulted from the negative attitude of many health officials. Field personnel were reluctant to report cases for fear of sanctions and criticism from their superiors. To overcome the problem, WHO instituted financial rewards for reporting cases. (The amount of the reward reached 1000 rupees by 1974. Compared with the average daily wage, this was a very substantial incentive; it was more than several months wages for many people.) Many people criticized the large amount that was paid extra to persons to do what they should do routinely anyway. But the reward system achieved results. The reward assessed not only the work of search workers but also the impact of the national publicity campaign. Cases could probably not be hidden for very long if everyone knew about the reward.

An unexpected problem arose from organizational arrangements that forced members into conflicting roles—those of surveillance *and* containment. When responsibility for finding cases was combined with responsibility for containment, the result was a certain role conflict. For this reason, the functions of surveillance and containment were separated organizationally. Henderson notes one of the practical problems that arose in developing an effective surveillance program:

> Most unexpected was the frequent failure in the development of the surveillance programme where responsibility for its development was entrusted to those also responsible for systematic vaccination activities. Daily concern to meet fixed vaccination targets mesmerized many into evaluating the success of the programme solely on this measurement.[9]

The campaign staff hammered constantly to improve the reporting system and data management. In this area the magnitude of the task was intimidating; two observations suggest the problem:

> The reporting efficiency couldn't have been more than 1 or 2 percent [in Uttar Pradesh]. . . . the Indians were sometimes deliberately hiding smallpox cases. Lower level officials who reported cases were blamed for inadequate vaccination. So it became easier not to report cases.[10]
> . . . they would not admit that they ever had smallpox. You weren't supposed to have smallpox. Government decrees would come down; There will be no smallpox! And these guys just would not report. [Some] people reporting cases were threatened with transfer or dismissal.[11]

Basically the same problem existed in other regions. In Indonesia, the fundamental problem was "the considerably incomplete reporting at village level." It was often found that village chiefs knew of cases, but did not report. Evidence suggested that "many outbreaks are reported only when the third or fourth generation of cases occur."[12]

Henderson observed, after a site visit to Rajasthan and Uttar Pradesh in 1971,

> The obvious and most urgent need of the program in India continues be in the area of reporting, surveillance and containment activities. Unless more current and accurate data are available at all levels, program planning is bound to continue to be seriously handicapped, coordination of activities between States and districts will be difficult or impossible, and the program itself must necessarily fail to reach the now foreseeable goal of eradication.
> . . . It was frequently noted that the civil authorities who are supposed

to report cases do not do so and that reporting of outbreaks is often very late.[13]

In general, paperwork was orchestrated carefully in order to record events so that strategy and tactics could be altered as needed to affect the outcome. As the program progressed, systems of cross-notification were developed, especially whenever outbreaks were traced to a source in neighboring country. This was important in controlling the spread of outbreaks, and was used with good results in Nepal, Bangladesh, and India. This was considered especially important by the headquarters staff. Foege observed that in the India campaign, over 100,000 people checked over 100 million houses in a very short period and in the process generated a mountain of paperwork. The experience made Foege "much less allergic to paperwork" because he could appreciate the value of controls and data under such circumstances.[14]

Henderson expressed even stronger reaction in assessing the progress in the India campaign in 1971: ". . . our principal disappointment this year has been the lack of progress thus far made by India in respect to improved reporting."[15]

More cases appeared to come to the notice of health authorities, but many were never recorded at national level. One state recorded 1,000 more cases than were recorded at the national level, and of course, 1,000 more than were reported to WHO.

> This deficit from a single state . . . amounts to fully 14 percent of all cases recorded in India this year and 4 percent of the world's total of cases. . . . Unless an effective reporting and surveillance programme is developed, there is no prospect whatsoever for a successful eradication programme.[16]

Brilliant describes the situation in India in 1971–72 as "working in the dark." The leadership of the smallpox program in New Delhi simply did not know at all accurately where the cases were or the magnitude of the disease. Many more months of patient demonstration and constant hammering on local and district health offices were required to make the reporting system credible as a useful tool in planning surveillance and containment.[17] When an active search strategy was first used in northern India in the autumn of 1973, the smallpox program was astonished by the result. During the week *before* the active search only 354 cases had been reported in 21 out of 55 districts in Uttar Pradesh. The week-long active search discovered 5,989 cases in 47 of the 55 districts and cases in 1,483 villages and 42 municipalities.[18] The search results clearly confirmed the problem of inadequate passive routine reporting and indicated the urgency of instituting regular active searches as a standard feature of the eradication campaign.

Writing after the eradication campaign had entered its fourth year, D. A. Henderson referred to other practical problems that the program had encountered.

> Other significant obstacles included national health authorities, wedded to the old mass vaccination concept, who could not comprehend the need for reporting; the academic idealists who were wholly confident that morbidity reporting was inevitably in error and who insisted that only a statistically correct sample survey could ever provide meaningful data; and the almost inevitably conservative statisticians who were highly agitated by the thought of concurrent use of and, if necessary revision of more rapidly collected morbidity data.[19]

Severe deficiencies in reporting cases were noted by Foster and his colleagues in Bangladesh. Sample surveys after the major epidemic in late 1971 indicated that only ten percent of the actual cases had been reported.

> This suppression of reporting dated back to the prewar mass vaccination programme when authorities considered a report of smallpox an admission of incomplete vaccination and actually punished the reporting health workers.[20]

Despite all these pleas, the government of India resisted changing the format of reports in 1971 so that smallpox data would be treated specially.[21] The emergency plan of 1974—a reorganization of health services— actually made the suppression of reporting a punishable offense.[22] Shortly thereafter, a reward for reporting was established. The Indian government finally recognized the importance of making the reporting of cases an action to be commended. Eventually even competition to report cases developed.

Some field team personnel reported, however, that in the epidemic stage, not much attention was paid to voluminous paperwork, except for the incidence report. Henderson's attitude was said to be "don't send reports—do the job!" and efforts were made to limit paper flow.[23]

Two fundamental questions relating to organizational philosophy, management approach, and political control of the smallpox eradication campaign were never fully resolved. The first of these questions is the matter of vertical, special purpose organizations versus integrated health care systems. This issue is discussed in further detail below. The second problem arose from the related issue of national (country) control of the specially focused smallpox eradication campaign.

Organizational Relationships

The latter issue, in general, was far simpler to resolve, in spite of a number of differences that arose between WHO and host countries or between CDC and (for example) the French *Service des Grandes Enfermies* in Gabon. Both in the international health community and among individual participants in the eradication campaign, there were sharp disagreements as to the extent to which host countries should control the program. There can be little doubt that in many instances the smallpox eradication campaign was delayed severely because of poor indigenous public health systems or because of slow-acting health authorities.

WHO's early policy papers regarding the organization of the smallpox campaign clearly envisioned it in terms of national programs:

> Though WHO gives assistance and advice, eradication campaigns are national programs and should be under the direction of an experienced senior medical officer designated by the government. A centralized and efficient administrative organization which should be responsible for all aspects of the campaign should be established.[24]

Of course, there was a sound practical basis for such policy. One overall strategy would not work, given the global scope of the smallpox eradication campaign. It was necessary to accommodate to diverse systems of health services in different countries, both in quality and scope. A further factor was the need to maximize use of existing health services in various countries because of the extremely limited budget of WHO for the campaign. In practice, such policy statements were far more difficult to implement. For various reasons, efforts to move the campaign rapidly were frustrated. India, for example, in 1971 resisted bringing in more consultants on the grounds that India had plenty of professionals.[25] Indeed, India may have had an adequate professional corps, but in the words of another participant in the India campaign,

> the medical structure was not only *not* effective in smallpox, it was counterproductive. The medical officers didn't get out of their clinics and into the villages, and the people who were the most useful and helpful in combating smallpox were the civil authorities, who tended to be more interested in what was really going on in the population at the village level. . . . Besides, we had been told time and time again by Indian officials that the villages in our areas had smallpox because the inhabitants were

ignorant and refused vaccination. . . . We found time and time again, as everyone who had worked there, that this assertion simply wasn't true. The people didn't resist vaccination, they resisted the *vaccinators*. The vaccinators were members of the Congress party, they were of the Brahman caste, they were hostile toward villagers who were either not Hindus or were of lower caste. They came in with a vicious, undiplomatic attitude and were physically abusive.[26]

Nicole Grasset was able finally to convince Prime Minister Indira Gandhi that autonomy for the smallpox campaign was essential. This was a major achievement for the Indian eradication program because it had suffered from constant diversion of its resources to other programs such as family planning.

The observation of one participant about the Indian campaign indicated the intimidating scope of the smallpox situation in India. The previous attitude among most epidemiologists was "let's do what we can, then get to India." By the time the Indian campaign commenced in earnest, surveillance-containment had proven itself. The dramatic success of the Indonesian campaign was highly persuasive to Indian health authorities. The Swedes came in with large donations of funds and gave the campaign an important boost at a critical time.[27]

William Foege commented that pride was a major motivation for the Indians because of their relatively well-developed health system. They felt that if Africa could beat smallpox, they could too.[28] Indian health planners also took note of the implementation of the surveillance-containment strategy in Indonesia, which shared many problems similar to India's: the strategy had been remarkably successful in Indonesia from 1969 to 1972.[29] Another participant describes the Indian system as "byzantine" but the people as bright.[30]

A vignette: Foege, a modest man (whom most people consider to be the originator of the surveillance-containment strategy as well as the hero of the West Africa and India campaigns) admits to being discouraged and doubtful only once in India in May 1974. An intimidating combination of circumstances caused that. This was the peak transmission period, hot, difficult to work in, just before the monsoons. Smallpox was increasing relentlessly. The explosion of India's first nuclear bomb had focused press attention on India, and the press played up the rise of smallpox outbreaks. Parliament was demanding explanations, a railroad strike disrupted movement of supplies to Bihar; in Putna, medical people struck so that over half the vaccinators quit work; M.D.s were to strike in June. In the midst of this discouraging situation, the health minister of Bihar lost faith in the surveillance strategy and wanted to go back to mass vaccination, demanding a public change of policy. However, he was persuaded to call a meeting of epidemiologists for counsel, and at that meeting, one person used a fire-fighting analogy to convince the minister. "If a house is afire in a village, the firefighters attack the fire, not the other houses in the village." The minister relented, gave more time, and the crisis passed. According to Foege, it was "all downhill" from that point. The attitudes of the people in general changed radically when the downturn started. "You can't work forever with failure."[31]

Generally, the objective was to have an independent campaign with health personnel detached from their regular jobs. The campaign was to work with local authorities in such a way as not to compromise local health programs.[32] But WHO advisers hammered on the importance of autonomy for the smallpox program. In Upper Volta, differences arose between the French health officials and CDC teams, the former not believing in delegation and use of locals.[33]

In Bangladesh, the question of organizational relationships created severe problems. Stanley Foster observed that the campaign was in "big trouble" because of the existence of three chains of authority and responsibility—a health chain, a malaria chain, and a civil surgeon chain. When Foster was able to convince the ministry, he redesigned the line of authority so that at each level a single person was responsible.[34] Others resorted to a system of "level jumping." In India, M.I.D. Sharma's approach was to

Go to the top. We level jumped and I could go to the minister of health, Karin Singh, whenever I felt like it. I would ring him up, or he would ring me, any time. . . . Singh usually was completely supportive of the program. He absorbed many of the pressures from elsewhere in the government. . . .[35]

Agreeing with Sharma, Brilliant notes how the organizational tactics of the smallpox team employed a "personal, persistent approach" to key personnel in government, politicians, bilateral donors, and philanthropists who in some cases were crucial to the campaign's success. He describes the nature of the operation as "an informal atmosphere, a group decision-making process, and an open, decentralized style."[36] In effect, an "informal leadership partnership" developed gradually as the "high command" for the smallpox eradication campaign in India.[37] This partnership amounted to an important extension of the use of counterparts which had been used in other WHO health programs.

As has been suggested, patterns of relations with host country health systems varied greatly. In West Africa, typically, the campaign approach was to beef up the *Service des Grandes Enfermies*. But in other areas, regular health programs suffered when people were pulled from them. Some programs were dying anyway (for example, malaria, because of growing mosquito resistance to DDT). In other countries, the smallpox campaign probably helped by strengthening health systems in general (although many in AID apparently think that the campaign retarded other health programs). In some areas, such as Bangladesh, an effort was made to meet the needs of other programs along with those of smallpox, and to assist in the transition from smallpox.[38] In India, at the height of the final (almost desperate) drive to control and eradicate smallpox in 1974, the director of the National Institute of Communicable Diseases (NICD) was freed from malaria control responsibilities in order to lead the smallpox eradication program full time. That decision was critical in the final eradication drive. The subsequent victory over smallpox left an experienced group of health officials ready to continue programs against malaria, diarrhea, blindness, vaccine-preventable diseases, and other health programs.[39]

In India, support from non-health organizations (general governmental administration) proved to be very important. District magistrates played a prominent part in Bihar when the large number of outbreaks exceeded the capacity of health officials. General administrators were crucial in achieving coordination with defense, railways, public sector organizations, and industry. Many voluntary organizations contributed by publishing health education materials and providing other materials to supplement government efforts.[40] As the Indian campaign progressed, so of course did the demand for funding and innovative financial management. Fund raising outside normal channels became an important source of support for the campaign. International agencies, governments, corporations, and private philanthropists were approached for assistance by WHO project staff. The Swedish International Development Agency (SIDA) made substantial contributions at critically important times. Tata Industries and other corporations provided cash and donations in kind as well as vital professional and organizational assistance. Civic groups such as the Lions and Rotary Club in India and groups such as OXFAM contributed financially and helped build support at the community level.

In terms of organizational structure, the WHO Manual for the most part was flexible in permitting necessary action and changes to meet circumstances to provide for cash payment, rewards, and a host of similar field situations. There is no question that Henderson and the smallpox eradication campaign had substantial autonomy. No small number of people in WHO today believe that the campaign bent many rules, but at least one high WHO official attributes the campaign style to the fact that Henderson was "a strong manager who eradicated mismanagement."[41] Many at WHO viewed the smallpox program negatively because it ran outside the regular WHO system.[42] Some even wondered fearfully (out of concern for job security), "What will we do if we eradicate smallpox?"[43] Some WHO officials were highly skeptical of the smallpox eradication campaign. One commented that if the India campaign were successful, he'd "eat a tire off a jeep." When the last case was reported, D. A. Henderson sent that person a jeep tire.[44]

Pragmatic management was the key to much of the campaign's success. According to one participant, WHO seemed to have lots of bureaucratic rules and procedures, but he tried to make the rules work for the smallpox campaign. This required a huge logistic effort. For example, the need for cash led to voluminous paperwork and often cash flowed simply on Henderson's assurance that funds were coming. The attitude, "either run a sloppy show or no show at all," seems a realistic view of the situation in Southeast Asia. Of course, there were losses and misappropriation, but not many relatively. Nicole Grasset, a WHO consultant in India, for example, was described as "one for cutting corners." The regional finance officer often had to cover a fait accompli, but it was "an act of faith well justified."[45] He saw himself as helping to cut corners where needed or in "mopping up" after a campaign. As an example, on one occasion, a program consultant appeared at the New Delhi regional WHO office on the way home to ask for pay. It was the first time he had been heard of by the regional office.[46] Another participant recalled,

> We got things done—I didn't look for rules. We talked with people, convinced them to make exceptions. We used the system to full advantage.[47]

Z. Jezek, who worked in the India campaign from 1971 to 1976 and in Somalia from 1976 to 1979, emphasized that WHO did not interfere unnecessarily with field operations and recognized that policies and programs had to be adapted to local conditions. The smallpox eradication campaign gave a boost to the effectiveness of the Indian health services by its "super-simplified methodology," so that the lowest level workers clearly understood their job. People could be motivated if clear, visible targets were set and methodology and technology kept simple. Jezek observed that sometimes European and American ideas about mobility, etc. were troublesome; he tried to use the habits and customs of locals whenever possible.[48]

There is little doubt that program procedures and operations in some areas were "allowed to shortcut or ignore some of the traditional steps in the health hierarchy." Mobile surveillance teams in Bangladesh are a prominent example. Typically, the teams were composed of health personnel withdrawn from their regular assignment. The special assignment gave members an "implied authority" which was "inconsistent with their strict civil service rank."

> This bastard authority and the special privileges of the surveillance teams— e.g., special travel subsidies, use of vehicles—might create enough resentment among local staff to hamper operations were it not for the presence of foreign advisors.[49]

Unfortunately, the vertical structure of the campaign left many field workers (who had enjoyed status, bonuses, cars, etc.) vulnerable after the campaign was over.[50]

Brilliant notes that the use of impact funds in the field, whereby health advisers carried large amounts of cash so as to be able to pay local expenses efficiently, created "substantial initial controversy" in WHO, which was not at all accustomed to such corner-cutting routines. But gradually, the WHO financial controllers understood and came to accept the necessary practice. The need to respond rapidly to changing circumstances eventually permeated the organization.[51]

Vertical vs. Horizontal Programs

One of the most difficult problems confronted by WHO is the question of the optimal organizational arrangement of its international health programs. More particularly, the issue revolves around whether health programs should be carried out by means of vertical, special purpose organizations or integrated into broad health care systems. The debate continues currently in WHO; indeed, it is a widely controversial issue not only in health but in management generally.

The smallpox eradication program, of course, functioned as a "vertical," or special and centrally-directed single-purpose organization. The sole mission of the program was the eradication of smallpox. (The West African campaign also included measles control in its mission, but WHO was involved only peripherally in that operation.) There was never any doubt or uncertainty about the program's objectives, and the clear goals (once the question of mass vaccination was resolved in favor of surveillance-containment) facilitated a single-minded focus for everyone concerned.

In WHO, the question tends to lead people to choose sides rather quickly. The issue is still somewhat emotional, suggesting that the smallpox eradication campaign created much controversy in the WHO bureaucracy. My own conclusion in this respect is that the smallpox campaign receives only grudging approval from many of those outside the campaign. Much of WHO often takes a negative view of the campaign, looking upon it as an example of *how not* to do things. Some in WHO still say, "the smallpox eradication campaign was successful, but they didn't do it the right way."[52]

On the side of vertical, special purpose organizations, one participant in the smallpox campaign concludes that neither WHO nor the less developed countries have learned what they should from the campaign. WHO might be better off to define problems more narrowly, rather than to announce goals such as "good health for everyone by 2000." This person went on to say that

> [WHO's] failure to do so may be due to people's wanting to be comfortable and not rock the boat. The organization strives for tranquility. It's a gentleman's club. WHO seems to be not goal-oriented.[53]

One WHO consultant observed that vertical programs are not in favor. But, ironically, the WHO Expanded Program on Immunization (EPI) and the Campaign Against Diarrheal Diseases (CDD)—both vertical, special programs—seem to be high priority programs and are considered likely to succeed. Others (horizontal, or integrated programs) such as malaria, family planning, and mental health probably won't succeed.[54] An assistant director-general saw nothing wrong with vertical programs when appropriate, but he would oppose another vertical program unless all factors were right. Most countries are too concerned with health maintenance programs to be ready for, say, a vertical malaria campaign.[55]

One participant in the Bangladesh campaign expressed strong opposition to another vertical disease control program. In some respects, he saw the campaign doing more damage than good. A large establishment was set up, but it could not be converted. It destroyed the careers of many people and overpaid many out of proportion. Careers were disrupted and the campaign subverted the regular health system. The same person also considered that it was outside pressure and money that made smallpox eradication the umber one priority in Bangladesh. He viewed many other diseases as far more destructive, but the feasibility of smallpox eradication gave it priority.[56] It should be noted that this view was distinctly in the minority, especially among participants in the campaign.

Looking back on the experience and evaluating the vertical organization of the campaign, D. A. Henderson observed that

> it made important contributions to the overall development of health services because, far from being separately or autonomously administered, it worked with and through the existing national health service structures and had to coordinate its activities with those of other programmes. The basic health services network, for instance, constituted the foundation of the disease-reporting structure, and in all countries this had to be greatly

improved by training and supervision in order to become effective and to provide the quick and accurate information on which the containment of smallpox outbreaks depended. The programme had targets and it provided supervision. Some may criticize it for being a so-called vertical programme but I believe it is a characteristic of successful programmes to have goals and necessary specialized management to attain these goals. Until other health programmes perform in a similar manner, I am afraid little progress will be made. Happily, however, some are beginning to do so.[57]

WHO Functions

The role of WHO in the smallpox eradication program was much broader than running the field campaigns. Besides its coordinative function, which became increasingly important after the conclusion of the successful effort in West Africa (run mainly by the CDC), the chief WHO contributions were in the direction of research activities, gathering of resources, identification of needs, and collection and dissemination of information on a global scale.

Research activities focused initially on the verification of certain basic assumptions regarding characteristics of smallpox (e.g., the absence of animal reservoirs of the virus) and laboratory control with respect to vaccine quality and production and diagnosis from specimens. Later, as the worldwide campaign successfully eradicated smallpox from country after country, the WHO research activities were concerned primarily with the certification of eradication by international commissions and surveillance regarding human monkeypox as well as operation of the rumor register for verification of reported cases of smallpox.

Recognizing the importance of accurate diagnosis of smallpox, WHO set about early to produce a set of teaching aids, including posters and slides showing smallpox and varicella at different stages of evolution of the rash. Laboratory diagnosis became more critical as the incidence of the disease dropped. So a network of diagnostic labs (CDC, Atlanta, and the Research Institute of Virus Preparations, Moscow) was developed, each of which was equipped to do three basic examinations for identification of the variola virus:

1. a microscopic smear examination
2. a gel precipitation test (This test proved to be of limited value because of its comparatively low sensitivity.)
3. virus isolation on the chorioallantoic membrane of chick embryo

A lab guide, *Guide to the Laboratory Diagnosis of Smallpox for Eradication Programmes* (1969), was prepared to describe in detail and pictorially each of these tests. "Unknown" specimens were distributed twice yearly to the labs to be sure they maintained competence.[58]

The campaign was supported by WHO collaborating centers (one in Atlanta, one in Moscow) for vaccine and diagnostic testing. Rapid laboratory backup significantly increased the efficacy of emergency measures. Specimens received in WHO from the field were dispatched immediately, with explanations for any delay. Rapid turn-around was the usual rule. Average times from date of receipt of specimens to dispatch of results to the field were as follows:

- seven days for initial potency and rapid stability test for vaccine samples
- three days for electron microscopic examination of pox virus particles
- seven days for virus isolation

The two laboratories investigated some 16,000 specimens from Asia and Africa during the campaign.[59] (See Figure 3.1.)

There is general agreement that WHO's presence was felt very little in West Africa or Brazil. It had essentially no operational control there. Communications for the Brazil campaign were primarily through PAHO, the Pan American Health Organization. Relations with WHO were mainly by means of personal contacts with Henderson. Some jealousy appeared to exist between PAHO and WHO.[60] But WHO did make two very important contributions in terms of using its good offices to gain entry of the United States into countries such as Congo Brazzaville and Guinea and providing critically needed funds for gasoline. The latter helped forge a link between WHO, CDC, and AID. Henderson is described virtually unanimously as doing an outstanding job as a diplomat and a fundraiser. One field officer called him "fantastically dedicated."[61] To a certain extent, he found it necessary to disassociate himself from the United States in order to be effective in his international WHO role.[62]

WHO is credited with doing a "bang-up" job in Zaire after 1970, Zaire being the first African country where surveillance-containment was used thoroughly. The world organization became highly influential in Asia, but only after completion of the West African campaign and shifting of U.S. efforts to Asia. Quick WHO response to the field was the case mainly in India, Bangladesh, Somalia, and Ethiopia. The vast majority of advisers and consultants continued to be CDC personnel.[63]

Once WHO's involvement in the Asian and East African campaigns intensified, the headquarters staff provided what is described generally as magnificent support. "The field got what it needed." There were frequent field visits by the staff, yet field teams enjoyed freedom to operate, with little second guessing by headquarters.[64] Flexibility was

FIGURE 3.1 Specimens Collected Worldwide and Tested by WHO Collaborating Laboratories, 1972-1979

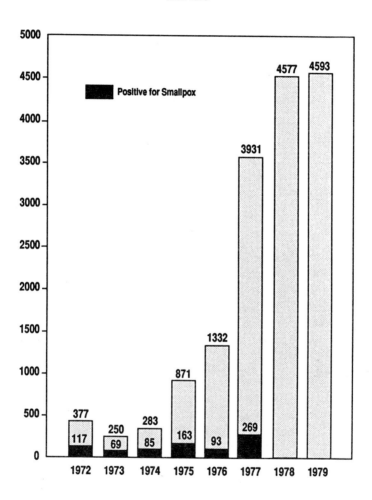

Source: WHO. The Global Eradication of Smallpox. (Geneva: WHO, 1980), p.56.

encouraged and the WHO headquarters was very supportive of this mode. The campaign was described by most participants as an operational program; getting things done rather than shuffling papers was the rule.[65]

In general, the interviews indicated that there were no insurmountable problems of organizational relationships. Basically, at least in the relation between WHO and CDC, there was mutual appreciation of the respective roles and the particular contributions that each organization could make. CDC continued to play an enormously important role in India and

Bangladesh, two of the most difficult areas in the campaign. Basically, CDC ran the West Africa program and had virtually complete responsibility. One person observed that CDC's "freewheeling" attitude "gave WHO fits," but such bureaucratic and political problems are inevitable.[66] There was some "jockeying" in the campaign for position and territory. Two senior officials, for example, referred to the CDC resentment of WHO's publishing a CDC smallpox eradication manual almost verbatim as a WHO publication, and in earlier publications almost ignoring the CDC role in West Africa.[67]

Some of the most difficult organizational relations appear to have existed between CDC and AID. The dual organizational structure between AID and CDC was an administrative nuisance; CDC apparently chafed under the routine AID treatment, although the country teams felt less pressure than the regional offices.[68] CDC was more "action-oriented" than AID, and many felt that "foot-dragging" and the detailed protocols of AID/State got in CDC's way. Again, however, such problems came mainly at the agency level rather than in the field. "Turf protection" clearly caused problems and these were aggravated by personalities.[69] Country ambassadors were generally supportive of the smallpox campaign because it gave them good press.[70] In the West Africa campaign, there were "tremendous difficulties" in getting country agreements signed; CDC had people recruited, trained, and waiting for AID to act.[71]

Some organizational arrangements in the West Africa campaign proved to be awkward and generally unproductive. For example, the regional office concept never worked effectively. The field teams were uncertain as to whether to use the channel through the Lagos regional office (the only such office created) or go directly to CDC headquarters. It soon became clear that CDC had the money and the power to decide and people began to deal directly with headquarters. The role gradually sorted itself out and after the first year the regional office did not push its supervisory role.[72]

As a means of coping with the uncertain regional office role, CDC created three zones in West Africa, each zone with a chief at CDC. Country directors then responded directly to zone chiefs. The regional office eventually handled personnel problems, difficulties between countries or zones, political representation, and evaluation.[73]

On occasion, CDC personnel may have been overly sensitive to the problems of AID, as Henderson once suggested pointedly. Dr. J. Michael Lane (CDC), writing about an assessment meeting, had expressed concern that AID might raise "possible charges of bias that we [CDC] might have against finding evidence that smallpox transmission is still going on."[74] Henderson responded,

I believe that you and CDC are all too sensitive to the AID nonsense of bias or charges of possible bias. Only AID could ferment the nonsense they have.[75]

Country Roles

Generally, there appeared to be no special problems that arose from the multinational composition of the eradication teams. William Foege saw one of the most difficult problems of all to be the persuasion of people at the top decisionmaking level. He described this as almost a "spiritual conversion," and it was tough until they became believers.[76] A large number of nations were represented in the campaign and in not a single instance did anyone express the feeling that any control came from outside WHO. "There was no big power competition in the smallpox campaign." (In a few situations, outsiders attempted to capitalize on big power rivalry, so as to embarrass one side or the other, as in the capture of a WHO helicopter in the Ogaden.)[77]

There does appear to have been some sensitivity with respect to the U.S. presence in the campaign. A "little jockeying" took place between WHO and CDC regarding the U.S. role, but most WHO publications clearly credit the United States for its major contributions. WHO, a political organization, attempted to emphasize the global nature of the smallpox eradication campaign.[78] Some people felt that Henderson, because he was an American, at times "soft-pedaled" the U.S. role.[79] Several participants criticized Henderson for publishing the CDC manual on smallpox eradication as a WHO publication without recognizing its origin. At a more personal level, one consultant recalls that to gain confidence, he first had to prove that he not a CIA agent.[80]

WHO and CDC relations with host countries varied considerably in their nature, style, and form. In the Brazil campaign, communications were mainly through PAHO. The campaign operated as a special vertical program in the Brazilian Ministry of Health. Different people took responsibility for various regions of Brazil and worked through state health departments. In general, Brazilians were cooperative and helpful. The effort was largely financed by Brazil, which produced its own vehicles and vaccine. The WHO presence was scarcely felt in Brazil, although PAHO representatives came from Washington fairly often.[81]

Country relations in the West Africa campaign were mixed. For example, Guinea had prior contact on a pilot measles project and a generally positive impression. But the government was somewhat wary of the "imperialist" United States. Guinea soon appreciated that the effort was strictly health, with no ulterior motives, and the government gave complete support to the operation.[82]

In Upper Volta, numerous problems plagued the campaign and many apparently arose from jealousy and resentment between CDC/AID and the French *Service des Grandes Enfermies*. Strong pressure came from the French to remove "eradication" from the program objectives because they had fought smallpox for years without complete success. Because the French already had a mandate on smallpox in Upper Volta, the CDC teams were phased into the SGE operation.[83] But a separate vertical organization was set up for smallpox and measles. Far more bitterness and hostility characterized relations in Upper Volta than in other countries.[84] In Sierra Leone, for example, which was under great pressure because of the large number of smallpox cases, the Ministry of Health was eager to begin the campaign and CDC personnel had to spend very little time "relating" to counterparts.[85]

In Bangladesh, assessing the initial problem of establishing surveillance, the WHO team found a very mixed situation in regard to reporting of smallpox cases. "Some subdivisions reported regularly, some reported infrequently, some reported rarely and a few had not reported for several months." When no reports were received from *thanas* (the basic administrative unit), this was interpreted to mean that there was no smallpox; actually it meant only that the *thana* had not reported.[86]

One of the first steps taken was to require all *thanas* to report weekly both to the Subdivisional Medical Office of Health (SDMOH) and to the national smallpox headquarters; this would be required even in the absence of smallpox. The concept of an outbreak was introduced, so that one infected village equaled one outbreak. When the government of Bangladesh agreed to active surveillance, 25 special surveillance teams supplemented the passive surveillance system with a highly mobile, active system.[87]

In Bangladesh, there was no national plan when the smallpox eradication began. The Bengali attitude, "do the needful," resulted in the creation of a national plan after several days of meetings and bargaining over policy.[88] The Emergency Plan of 1974 provided for a strictly vertical program structure for the eradication campaign. The former "organization jumble" with confusing lines of authority was replaced by a clear hierarchy from national headquarters through area smallpox officers (ASO) to *thana* smallpox officers (TSO) to resident supervisors (RS). Bangladesh was divided into areas, each assigned to an ASO. The ASO designated one person to be the TSO in each *thana*. The TSO was required to send a telegraphic report each week to the ASO and national headquarters on the status of smallpox in the *thana*. Smallpox occurrence was to be treated as an emergency, and once a case occurred a family welfare worker would take over as resident supervisor in the infected village, remaining until relieved. Release would come only after verification by a surveillance team member, a WHO advisor, an ASO, or the TSO that 42 days had elapsed without a new case. Vaccination was done by young men and women of the village itself, hired, trained, and supervised by the resident supervisor. Fixed inspection schedules were established.[89]

The global WHO system functions through a system of regional offices and this regionalization affects the nature of health programs in the region. The regional office director is elected by the countries of the region, and the director's authority is almost total, subject to general direction by the World Health Assembly. Of course, some regional offices are more influential than others and in the case of India and Bangladesh, the campaigns had to operate through the Southeast Asia Regional Office. Funds passed through and were accounted for by the regional office. This was a "difficult balancing act" for Henderson and WHO headquarters between the global effort and the regional offices.

Formally, of course, the regional office director was in charge.[90] Henderson relied heavily on the regional office, using feedback and contact to stay in touch with the overall operation. He was adept at maintaining good relations with the people who mattered. For example, almost all relations with Tata Industries, which provided major support for the campaign, were through Henderson. There were many problems with health ministries, over such matters as interpretation of agreements, but overall the government was committed strongly and made little difficulty.[91]

However, at times, the national health service could not cope. For example, in Bihar state at the peak of smallpox incidence in 1974, supplies and personnel were not adequate. The WHO consultant in Bihar moved around the district to mobilize private organizations and to make appeals. In two weeks, he had enlisted sufficient aid to create ten teams and employ 100 vaccinators.[92]

Local team practices regarding the most effective administrative arrangements varied substantially from place to place. In Uttar Pradesh, the campaign worked closely with the government. In Bihar, the independent system was set up. Each district typically had a medical officer and deputy medical officer, with generally a paramedical assistant who was most important in keeping programs moving—the "eyes and ears" of the operation. The typical initial approach was to size up the situation and resources for dealing with it, and visit areas of the greatest problems, checking for active cases and containment effectiveness. The next phase was search, broadening the radius from one to five to ten miles. Watchguards were used to control entrances to infected houses.[93] Sometimes control problems arose from reporting of other rash diseases such as chickenpox and measles, and workers sometimes gave vitamins or other pills for psychological purposes when reported cases were not smallpox.

On occasion, field teams were plagued by rumors that they were performing vasectomies instead of vaccinations.[94]

In Bihar state, the WHO officer, having been told that he had complete freedom to operate as necessary in the state ("the district is in your hands") changed strategy as and when necessary in the district. The regional office had instructed the teams to use "ring vaccination." This was resisted by local health authorities and some district officers paid no attention to reports of smallpox outbreaks. The WHO consultant did not inform local authorities he was coming, in order to check the local situation independently. He started active search, and although the case incidence for his district was the highest, he was encouraged, because some local officers had been reporting zero cases when outbreaks were obvious. The ten new teams made a great difference in detection and by July 1974, Bihar became the first smallpox-free state.[95]

Field workers also were adept at devising means for coping with the uncertainty of campaign existence. Sometimes field team personnel deliberately sent dummy specimens such as chickenpox to the analysis laboratories in order to check on their performance and accuracy.[96] In Bangladesh, in order to justify the payment of workers that were needed (above the rate limited by the government), non-existent villages were created to support the receipt for funds. A substantial number of these appear in the final reports of infected villages, but they do not exist. This action was rationalized on the grounds that money was needed and there was no other way.[97]

In Somalia, the last battle of the global campaign, the WHO smallpox eradication unit insisted on a strong central head with every aspect of the operation working through him. Logistics were squared away and the basic building blocks erected first. The system was set up completely before any epidemiologists started work. The smallpox eradication campaign came in from the outside and did the job. The program basically was independent of the health ministry of Somalia.[98]

Respondents agreed virtually unanimously that field requests were given top priority by headquarters, both CDC and WHO. This was very important and provided a tremendous morale boost to the field. On occasion even meetings with the WHO director-general were cancelled in order to handle field problems. The relationship was two-way; Henderson observed that most good ideas came from the field.[99] From a CDC headquarters perspective, most problems were management and logistics problems rather than medical. The main difficulties were communications, the logistics of shipping and lead time, and vehicle maintenance. Funding was not a serious problem.[100]

Basic logistic problems were a constant fact of life in most of the country campaigns. Peter Crippen recalled from Bangladesh,

Transportation in most of Bangladesh is difficult, tiring, and incredibly slow. The journey from Dacca to Faridpur—a distance of eighty miles—requires five hours by car. The journey from Madaripur to Goshairat (two towns in Faridpur District)—a distance of thirty miles—requires five hours by speedboat. The journey from Shibchar to Kalu Bhayer Kandi—a distance of nine miles—requires three hours on foot. There are four things to remember: have enough money to hire whatever transport you need; keep in mind that if people live there, there must be *some* way to get there; if you're riding, take along a book; if you're walking, don't take anything.[101]

Personnel Administration

For an international effort of the dimensions of the global smallpox eradication campaign, there were remarkably few problems of personnel administration. During the twelve year period of the campaign after 1967, 687 field epidemiologists and administrators provided by WHO from 73 countries participated in the program; at any one time no more than 150 WHO staff members were working in the campaign.[102]

To a large extent, the personnel recruitment network was personal and casual—no extensive testing was required. A kind of "old-boy" network was employed to check out the people, almost all of whom had overseas experience. The WHO bureaucracy did not take well to this, although the WHO personnel office seemed glad to be relieved of some of the recruitment problems and delegated as much responsibility as possible to the smallpox eradication unit. In the early stages, when the principal concern was with problems such as vaccine quality, the most important criterion was technical competence. Later, when the field campaign intensified and accelerated, preference was given to the people with overseas experience (Peace Corps volunteers, etc.).[103]

As a rule, consultants for the smallpox campaign were much younger than normal for WHO. Complications of recruitment depended largely on the nationality of consultants. The most difficult appointments were for East Europeans and Soviet Union consultants; the easiest were from the United Kingdom and France. Consultants from the United States also were easy to process; they would often head for duty posts without government approval or paperwork. Sometimes the visa process was bypassed but this was dangerous because host governments had to agree to accept consultants.[104]

The WHO personnel office view was that the personnel administration system operated as normal in the processing of appointments. The smallpox eradication campaign was given priority, but its work was just part of the usual personnel work (even though for the campaign "it was everything. Everything had to be done yesterday."). On occasion recruitment outran paperwork and this had to catch up later.[105]

Most respondents agreed that the campaign suffered relatively few personnel problems. Very few people proved unsuitable for overseas work. One person, for example, was not sensitive to the host country's needs and was terminated early.[106] Another person, who simply could not adjust to Africa, was reassigned to CDC, where he did a good job.[107] Another respondent commented, "not more than five out of 250 epidemiologists were failures" in the Bangladesh campaign.[108] There were no serious problems in Sierra Leone, but two "grossly inappropriate" people were sent home.[109]

Consultants played a major role in the campaign. They were often able to accomplish much quickly and their independence, outside authority, and prestige were important. Thus careful management of consultants was a critical factor in the campaign's success.[110] For the West and Central Africa Smallpox Eradication and Measles Control Program, training for U.S. technicians was provided at the NCDC in Atlanta. Specialized training was given in public health, methodology, smallpox eradication and measles control, and program management and operations. Further training was provided in the project countries, including practical instruction in operation and repair of jet injectors, clinical diagnosis of smallpox and measles, vaccine handling, assessment and surveillance, and related matters.[111]

As the campaign developed, it became increasingly clear that *the effort was a management operation as much as it was epidemiologic.* For this reason, the concept of public health advisers (PHA) received more and more attention and another important factor in the campaign's achievements was the use of such personnel. The idea was formulated in the 1940's, when CDC began to use qualified management people to do some of the grass roots epidemiologic work, especially in venereal disease control. Such use expanded greatly in the 1960's. Eventually public health advisers became a major element in the West Africa campaign. Very often managerial expertise proved more important than medical knowledge. It soon became clear that PHA's could handle most epidemiologic problems as well and in some areas M.D.'s reported to the public health advisers. Upon the division of West Africa by CDC into three areas, PHA's became chiefs of operations for two of the areas.[112]

Generally, the concept worked well. Some problems of status arose in West Africa but for the most part, non-medical personnel were less threatening to local M.D.'s. Most PHA's became well respected for their work.[113] Jezek recalls that people were too busy in India and Somalia to worry about status.[114] Brilliant observes that in India the use of operations officers, most of whom were PHA's from the CDC, was an important factor in the effective working of the logistic system in the campaign.[115]

Another potential difficulty—the multinational character of the campaign—never proved to be a serious problem. About 22 nationalities worked in the Bangladesh campaign with no serious difficulty. There were some isolated problems. In 1977, for example, Americans were not welcome in Somalia. Some governments were concerned about security in regard to Soviet consultants and some Russians were described as insensitive toward Third World people and "really racists."[116] Overall, however, multinational groups functioned very effectively. The Indian campaign included participants from the following nations: Afghanistan, Australia, Austria, Belize, Bolivia, Brazil, Canada, Czechoslovakia, Denmark, Ethiopia, France, Ghana, Indonesia, Japan, Mexico, Nepal, the Netherlands, Norway, Poland, Romania, Singapore, Sri Lanka, Sweden, Switzerland, the United Kingdom, the United States, the USSR, West Germany, Yemen, and Yugoslavia. Jezek observed that questions of nationality never arose at the field level.[117]

Clearly, the campaign leaders saw the choice of good people to be an absolutely critical factor. William Foege, in discussing candidates with referees who knew them, always kept two central questions in mind: first, how well does the candidate work with other cultures (minorities, women, subordinates, etc.) in his or her *own* culture? and second, does the candidate have a positive approach to life? (As Foege observed, "One should not send a pessimist to India!"[118]) Henderson, in filling key posts, was extremely careful to get people in whom he had confidence.[119]

No small number of persons motivated by idealism were attracted to the campaign. One CDC specialist saw the campaign as "historically intriguing" and "idealistically appealing."[120] But their idealism was tempered by the hard-headed realism essential for survival and success in field operations. One consultant recalls being horrified not only by smallpox cases, but by India itself. But he was able to accept this and go about the job. Nevertheless, "the experience became almost a religious experience."[121] To another participant, the spirit of comraderie that characterized the campaign reflected "human effort at its best."[122]

In the following chapter, the focus shifts to an examination of the process through which the smallpox campaign organization learned from experience and incorporated that learning into its strategy.

Notes

1. Interview, Jock Copland (WHO), 4 November 1981.
2. Donald A. Henderson, "Smallpox Shows the Way," *World Health* (March 1977), 25.
3. Interview, John Wickett (WHO), 2 December 1981.
4. D. A. Henderson, "Surveillance of Smallpox," WHO/SE/75.76, 8.

5. Donald A. Henderson, "The Eradication of Smallpox." 235 *Scientific American* (October 1976), 30.

6. R. N. Basu, "Smallpox Surveillance Status in India." 6 *Journal of Communicable Diseases* (1974), 974 as cited by Brilliant. *The Management of Smallpox Eradication in India,* p. 21.

7. D. A. Henderson, "Surveillance of Smallpox," WHO/SE/75.76, pp. 7–8.

8. H. M. Gelfand, "A Critical Examination of the Indian Smallpox Eradication Program," 56 *American Journal of Public Health* (1966), 1644, as cited in Lawrence B. Brilliant, *The Management of Smallpox Eradication in India,* p. 13.

9. D. A. Henderson, "Epidemiology in the Global Eradication of Smallpox." 1 *International Journal of Epidemiology* (Spring 1972), 27.

10. William H. Foege (CDC) as quoted by Shurkin, *The Invisible Fire,* p. 319.

11. John Wickett (WHO) as quoted by *ibid.,* p. 319–320.

12. P. A. Koswara, N. K. Rai, B. Wongsokusumo, I. Arita, V. Borg-Groch, A. Oles, "Report of an assessment of the smallpox eradication projects in Java and Bali, by a Joint Government of Indonesia/WHO Team, June 1969." SEA/Smallpox/31, 27 October 1969, p. 6.

13. D. A. Henderson, "Report on Visit to Smallpox Eradication Programs in Rajasthan and Uttar Pradesh, India, 5–20 April 1971," SEA/Smallpox/51, pp. 1–2.

14. Interview, William Foege (CDC), 13 May 1981.

15. D. A. Henderson. "Proceeding of the Inter-regional Seminar on Surveillance and Assessment in Smallpox Eradication, New Delhi, 30 November–5 December 1970," WHO/SE/71.30, p. 7.

16. *Ibid.,* p. 7.

17. Brilliant, *The Management of Smallpox Eradication in India,* pp. 21–26.

18. WHO. *The Global Eradication of Smallpox* (Geneva: WHO, 1980), p. 34.

19. D. A. Henderson, "Epidemiology in the Global Eradication of Smallpox." 1 *International Journal of Epidemiology* (Spring 1971), 27.

20. S. O. Foster, N. A. Ward, A. K. Joarder, N. Arnt, D. Tarantola, M. Rahman, and K. Hughes, "Smallpox Surveillance in Bangladesh: I–Development of Surveillance Containment Strategy," 9 *International Journal of Epidemiology* (1980), 329.

21. Interview, Joel Breman (CDC), 6 May 1981.

22. S. O. Foster *et al.,* "Smallpox Surveillance in Bangladesh," p. 330.

23. Interview, A. I. Gromyko (WHO), 20 November 1981.

24. "Organization of a Smallpox Eradication Campaign," WHO/Smallpox/20, 25 May 1964, p. 2.

25. Interview, Joel Breman (CDC), 6 May 1981.

26. J. Michael Lane, as quoted by Shurkin. *The Invisible Fire,* pp. 318–319.

27. Interview, Jock Copland (WHO), 4 November 1981.

28. Interview, William Foege (CDC), 13 May 1981.

29. Brilliant, *The Management of Smallpox Eradication in India,* pp. 16–17.

30. Interview, Jay Friedman (CDC), 12 May 1981.

31. Interview, William Foege (CDC), 13 May 1981.
32. Interview, Joel Breman (CDC), 6 May 1981.
33. Interview, Tom Leonard, (CDC), 12 May 1981.
34. Shurkin, *The Invisible Fire,* p. 358.
35. *Ibid.,* p. 327.
36. Brilliant, *The Management of Smallpox Eradication in India,* p. 93.
37. *Ibid.,* p. 96.
38. Interview, J. Michael Lane (CDC), 15 May 1981.
39. Brilliant, *The Management of Smallpox Eradication in India,* p. 52.
40. R. N. Basu, WHO draft document n.d. (1981?).
41. Interview, I. D. Ladnyi (WHO), 20 November 1981.
42. Interview, Donald R. Hopkins (CDC), 6 May 1981.
43. Confidential interview No. 3 (WHO).
44. Interview, William Watson (CDC), 13 May 1981.
45. Interview, A. J. R. Taylor (WHO), 2 December 1981.
46. *Ibid.*
47. Interview, John Wickett (WHO), 2 December 1981.
48. Interview, Z. Jezek (WHO), 15 December 1981.
49. P. H. Crippen, "Public Health Administration in a Developing Country—Major Problems Observed in Bangladesh." Unpublished manuscript, p. 4.
50. Interview, Peter H. Crippen (Indiana State Board of Health), 17 August 1978.
51. Brilliant, *The Management of Smallpox Eradication in India,* p. 113.
52. Interview, John Wickett (WHO), 2 December 1981.
53. Confidential interview (CDC), No. 4.
54. Interview, R. C. Hogan (WHO), 6 October 1981.
55. Interview, I. D. Ladnyi, (WHO), 20 November 1981.
56. Interview, Stanley Music (CDC), 13 May 1981.
57. "Smallpox Eradication: A WHO Success Story." Forum Interview with Donald A. Henderson. 8 *World Health Forum* (1987).
58. "Smallpox Eradication: The First Significant Results." 23 *WHO Chronicle* (1969), 476.
59. WHO Doc. CDS/Mtg./WP/81/35, p. 2.
60. Interview, Leo Morris (CDC), 13 May 1981.
61. Interview, Z. Jezek (WHO), 15 December 1981.
62. Interview, J. Michael Lane (CDC), 15 May 1981.
63. *Ibid.*
64. Interview, Stanley Foster (CDC), 7 May 1981.
65. Interview, Joel Breman (CDC), 6 May 1981.
66. Interview, William Watson (CDC), 12 May 1981.
67. Interviews, Donald Hopkins (CDC), 6 May 1981, and J. Donald Millar (CDC), 15 May 1981.
68. Interview, R. H. Henderson (WHO), 6 October 1981.
69. Interview, James Hicks (CDC), 12 May 1981.
70. Interview, J. Michael Lane (CDC), 15 May 1981.
71. Interview, J. Donald Millar (CDC), 15 May 1981.

72. Interview, R. C. Hogan (WHO), 6 October 1981.
73. Interview, J. Donald Millar (CDC), 15 May 1981.
74. Letter, J. Michael Lane (CDC) to D. A. Henderson (WHO), 13 August 1974.
75. Letter, D. A. Henderson (WHO) to J. Michael Lane (CDC), 23 August 1974.
76. Interview, William Foege (CDC), 12 May 1981.
77. Interview, A. I. Gromyko (WHO), 20 November 1981.
78. Interview, Joel Breman (CDC), 6 May 1981.
79. Interview, Jock Copland (WHO), 4 November 1981.
80. Interview, Joel Breman (CDC), 6 May 1981.
81. Interview, Leo Morris (WHO), 13 May 1982.
82. Interview, Joel Breman (CDC), 6 May 1981.
83. Interview, R. H. Henderson (WHO), 6 October 1981.
84. Interview, Tom Leonard (CDC), 12 May 1981.
85. Interview, Donald R. Hopkins, 6 May 1981.
86. Stanley I. Music, "Smallpox Eradication in Bangladesh: Reflections of an Epidemiologist," unpublished dissertation, London School of Hygiene and Tropical Medicine (1976), pp. 16–18.
87. *Ibid.,* pp. 18–21.
88. Interview, Stanley I. Music (CDC), 13 May 1981.
89. Stanley I. Music, "Smallpox Eradication in Bangladesh: Reflections of an Epidemiologist," pp. 38–41.
90. Interview, A. J. R. Taylor (WHO), 2 December 1981.
91. *Ibid.*
92. Interview, A. I. Gromyko (WHO), 20 November 1981.
93. Interview, Walter Orenstein (CDC), 8 May 1981.
94. *Ibid.*
95. Interview, A. I. Gromyko (WHO), 20 November 1981.
96. Interview, Mary Guinan (CDC), 15 May 1981.
97. Interview, Stanley I. Music (CDC), 13 May 1981.
98. Interview, John Wickett (WHO), 2 December 1981.
99. Interview, Joel Breman (CDC), 6 May 1981.
100. Interview, Billy Griggs (CDC), 6 May 1981.
101. P. H. Crippen, "Public Health Administration in a Developing Country: Major Problems Observed in Bangladesh." Unpublished manuscript, 1978(?).
102. Joel G. Breman and Isao Arita, "The Confirmation and Maintenance of Smallpox Eradication," 303 *New England Journal of Medicine* (November 27, 1980), 1264.
103. Interviews, Joel Breman (CDC), 6 May 1981, and Jock Copland (WHO), 4 November 1981.
104. Interview, Margaret Prandle (WHO), 4 December 1981.
105. *Ibid.*
106. Interview, Joel Breman (CDC), 6 May 1981.
107. Interview, James Hicks (CDC), 12 May 1981.
108. Interview, Stanley Foster (CDC), 7 May 1981.

109. Interview, Donald Hopkins (CDC), 6 May 1981.
110. Interview, Joel Breman (CDC), 8 May 1981.
111. James W. Hicks, "A Review of West African Operations: Methods and Tactics." *The SEP Report,* Vol. 4 (January 1970), p. 193.
112. Interview, James Hicks (CDC), 12 May 1981; R. C. Hogan (WHO), 6 October 1981; Donald R. Hopkins (CDC), 6 May 1981.
113. At least two WHO programs, the Expanded Program on Immunization (EPI) and Control of Diarrheoc Diseases (CDD) use the PHA concept currently.
114. Interview, Z. Jezek (WHO), 15 December 1981.
115. Brilliant, *The Management of Smallpox Eradication in India,* p. 100.
116. Confidential interview No. 5.
117. Interview, Z. Jezek (WHO), 15 December 1981.
118. Interview, William Foege (CDC), 13 May 1981.
119. Interview, Ralph H. Henderson (WHO), 6 October 1981.
120. Interview, Mary Guinan (CDC), 15 May 1981.
121. Interview, Walter Orenstein (CDC), 8 May 1981.
122. Interview, Ralph H. Henderson (WHO), 6 October 1981.

4

Organizational Learning

The global strategy for the eradication of smallpox is based on the fact that no nonhuman reservoir exists for smallpox, and therefore smallpox will cease to exist altogether once the last human case had occurred.
—Axnick and Lane (1972)

Foege is the hero.
—Mary Guinan, 15 May 1981

To understand the smallpox eradication campaign, we must give major attention to the matter of organizational learning. The concept may be defined in various ways. For my purposes, it refers to the organization's learning from continuing experience and incorporating that learning into the design of effective control devices and management strategies. The concept refers also to the organization's sensitivity and receptivity to a wide variety of ideas, inputs, and information. The organization has "learned" when a mismatch between intentions and results is detected and corrected. As Chris Argyris observed, "double-loop learning" occurs when "changes are made in the basic assumptions and policies of the unit."[1] "Organizational learning" is a short-hand concept referring to learning by members of organizations who in turn may modify the organizational framework, relationship, rules, and communication networks. Such aspects are crucially important because they serve to condition, facilitate, restrict, and sometimes prevent the learning and adaptive process.

In retrospect, it appears that the flexible mode of management adopted by the small staff in WHO who directed the campaign provided a felicitous environment for organizational learning and innovation.

Essentially problem-solvers, they viewed themselves as catalysts rather than as controllers. They understood from the onset that experimental learning offered the only possibility for success. They avoided formalized programming, opting instead for innovation, flexibility, communication, and experiment, by means of a number of deliberate policies and mechanisms.

They recruited people with practical field experience in epidemiology (as opposed to previous work with smallpox *per se*). They sought people with reputations for adaptability, imagination, and hard work. They preferred younger people, assuming they would be more receptive to new approaches and ideas.[2]

The flexible, open approach equipped the Smallpox Eradication Unit to respond more readily to challenges of problem definition and changes in tactics and strategy.

Problem Definition

At all stages of the eradication campaign, how the problem was defined proved to be critically important. Major shifts in strategy and the plan of attack followed a redefinition of the problem. Thus careful attention must be given to how the relevant organizations arrived at the original working definition of the problem. On what evidence was the definition based, and on what ground was the consensus achieved to attack the problem? To what extent did various considerations—scientific, economic, political—enter into the process of decision making? In retrospect, what conclusions may be drawn regarding the adequacy and soundness of the evidence?

In 1966, past experience in epidemiology and particularly in both successful and unsuccessful programs to control smallpox defined the problem facing WHO as essentially one of mass vaccination of people in endemic areas. Such programs in Western Europe, North America, Japan, and other areas, for all practical purposes, had eradicated smallpox. There is little doubt that, in general, the dominant thinking in the pre-1970 period favored mass vaccination as the principal strategy of smallpox control. As Brilliant observes in his study of the Indian campaign,

The concept of "herd immunity" dominated smallpox eradicators' thinking at the time. Basically, this meant that if enough people in a community were vaccinated and therefore immune to smallpox the disease could not perpetuate itself through the "herd" of people in that community. WHO as well as many governments stressed high vaccination coverage as the key to interruption of transmission.[3]

A 1966 report by the WHO director-general, as well as the strategy outlined in Figure 4.1, reflects such thinking:

Eradication can be accomplished in a comparatively simple and straightforward manner by rendering immune, through vaccination, a sufficiently large proportion of the population so that transmission is interrupted. *In*

FIGURE 4.1 Phases in the Smallpox Eradication Programme

	Attack Phase (Phase I)	Consolidation Phase (Phase 2)	Maintenance Phase (Phase 3)
Type of Vaccination	Systematic Mass Vaccination	Continuing Maintenance Vaccination	Continuing Matintenance Vaccination
Surveillance	*Reporting* Establishment of prompt and regular reporting of smallpox by all existing health facilities.	*Reporting* Extension of case detection system to assure that all suspected smallpox cases are reported.	*Reporting* Continuation of case detection system to ensure that all suspected cases are reported.
	Field Investigations Epidemiological investigation of major outbreaks throughout the country and of all cases in areas where systematic mass vaccination has been carried out.	*Field Investigations* Prompt epidemiological investigation of all cases to establish sources of infection and to exclude the possibility of unreported cases.	*Field Investigations* Each case investigated as an emergency by an epidemiologist.
Laboratory	Establishment of techniques and methods for the submission and examination of specimens for confirmation of diagnosis.	Specimens studied from isolated cases and representative samples from each outbreak	Specimens studied from every suspect case.
Containment	Localized, intensive vaccination in communities where outbreaks occur. Isolation of cases if feasible and disinfection.	Vaccination and observation of case contacts. Isolation of cases and appropriate disinfection. Localized, intensive vaccination in community.	Vaccination and and observation of case contacts. Isolation of cases and appropriate disinfection. Localized, intensive vaccination in community.
Criteria	Smallpox endemic with more than 5 cases per 100,000 population annually *and* with less than 80% of population showing primary vaccination scars.	Incidence less than 5 cases per 100,000 population annually *and* with over 80% of population showing primary vaccination scars.	Country free from endemic smallpox for more than 2 years, but geographically situated in an endemic continental area.

Source: 22 WHO Chronicle (1968), p. 361.

a highly endemic area this requires almost 100 percent coverage of the population. [emphasis added][4]

The rarity of outbreaks of the disease in the industrialized countries appeared to confirm the validity of that strategy. Vast sums of money had been expended over long periods in those countries to protect people against importation of the smallpox virus from infected areas. The policy choice of mass vaccination as a strategy seemed further supported, from the perspective of 1967, by tests conducted in 1964 and 1967 on the island of Tonga. Although the tests on Tonga had different objectives— the object actually was to test the efficacy of jet injection of vaccine and the duration of immunity conferred—the effectiveness of that experiment as well as other evidence appeared to lead logically to a strategy of worldwide mass vaccination in infected areas.

In fact, the Tonga tests were only one of a series of studies carried out by the Communicable Disease Center (CDC) in the 1960s, primarily to test the efficacy of vaccination by intradermal jet injection. Studies done in the United States, Jamaica, and Brazil, as well as Tonga, all led to the conclusion that jet injection was both safe and efficacious for primary vaccination and revaccination, when proper vaccines were used.[5]

Here again, it must be emphasized, although the objective of these studies was mainly to test jet injection, the logical inference was that jet injection was a valuable tool that would facilitate mass vaccination, and therefore mass vaccination appeared more feasible as the basis for a worldwide eradication campaign.

One might question—in hindsight—whether the sample size was adequate or whether experience in relatively small, highly limited, and essentially insulated environments such as Tonga could be transferred to projects worldwide in scope. Likewise, the apparent success of long-continued mass vaccination programs in North America and Europe, under far better controlled conditions, may have led to unjustified conclusions. A more careful review would have shown that mass vaccination was not accepted as a strategy in some countries, notably the United Kingdom. Similarly, the failure of the sporadic, underfunded, uncoordinated WHO program which began in 1959 influenced the choice of a mass vaccination policy in 1966. Logically, or at least one might reasonably conclude, the 1959 campaign failed (in large part) because the vaccination was not sufficiently mass-based, and a more thorough campaign of mass vaccination might succeed.

Jet injection was used for the first time in a national eradication program in Brazil in 1965, with very effective results. Several advantages of the technique were apparent from the Brazilian experience. These included reduction in manpower needs, reduction in transportation needs, increased efficiency of vaccination, and reduction in vaccine needs. It was calculated that the per vaccination cost for the jet injector campaign in Macapá, $0.022, was less than one-third of the costs of the multiple pressure campaign in Belém.[6] Such results lent support to a strategy of mass vaccination.

The point is that the policy choice of 1966 *appeared* at the time to be based upon logical evaluation of reasonably convincing experience, empirical tests, and demonstrated success. Accordingly, the problem was defined in terms of mass vaccination, and the smallpox eradication campaign commenced in 1967 with that basic strategy.

As the eradication campaign progressed, the effectiveness of the original eradication strategy came into question as apparently insurmountable problems arose. The program in Nigeria had continued an earlier joint effort of the Communicable Disease Center (CDC) and the U.S. Agency for International Development (AID) started in 1966. The objective of that program was to vaccinate 80 percent of the population over a three year period. However, in Western Nigeria, in spite of the fact that over 90 percent of the population had been vaccinated, another smallpox outbreak occurred, apparently originating in a religious group which had resisted vaccination. Delay in delivery of supplies forced a change in tactics. Such challenges led to a new strategic approach in place of the original strategy of mass vaccination. That critical shift in strategy, however, required a basic redefinition of the problem, organizational learning, and innovation to manage the new strategies as well as technological developments.

The Genesis of Surveillance and Containment

The Nigerian outbreaks, almost out of necessity, led to the adoption of a new strategy—surveillance and containment. In this approach, a reporting network was established—using whatever radio facilities were available—to insure quick pinpointing of new cases. Containment teams quickly moved to areas of outbreaks, isolating infected persons, and rapidly vaccinated entire villages of people. It was discovered that such rapid containment could break the transmission chain of smallpox, even where less than half the population had been vaccinated.

The new approach of surveillance and containment proved to be the foundation of the successful worldwide campaign. Its adoption was followed by dramatic decreases in the number of endemic countries. By 1973, only six countries were classified as endemic—but those six countries alone contained over 700 million people.

To appreciate the incremental development of the surveillance-containment strategy, we must examine further the background of the situation leading to adoption of the strategy as well as generally accepted epidemiological approaches to smallpox. The type of organizational learning exemplified by the smallpox eradication campaign raises important questions about our capability for rational decisionmaking, the application of knowledge, information retrieval systems, and technological innovation and diffusion. In addition, such major strategy shifts are likely to raise questions of ownership or authorship that may be organizationally disruptive, as well as problems of control and politics.

An examination of the WHO decision to undertake a smallpox eradication campaign clearly reveals a commitment to mass vaccination as the central epidemiological strategy. Preliminary papers issued by WHO to guide the organization of smallpox eradication services for the 1959 campaign envisioned mass vaccination as the chief means of attaining eradication.[7]

It is now generally agreed that if 80 percent of the population—that is, 80 percent of each and every sector of the population—is successfully vaccinated within a time period of five years, smallpox will die out.[8]

The strategy for the 1966 campaign showed an even stronger commitment to mass vaccination.

The aim of a national eradication campaign should be to vaccinate 100 percent of the population of the country. Experience has shown that a target of vaccinating 80 percent of each segment of the population has been found in practice to be unsatisfactory in certain cases.[9]

This strategy was based largely on the 1964 report of the WHO Expert Committee on Smallpox. The Committee proposed what Henderson was later to call the "impossible solution": vaccinate 100 percent of the population.[10]

Likewise, the WHO plan of operation for the global campaign called for vaccination of the entire population within as short a time as possible and, if possible, within three years. (Surveillance was discussed as an epidemiologic tactic but not emphasized.)[11] At the Ninth International Congress for Microbiology in Moscow, in July 1966, much of the discussion concerned the implications of "eradication" of disease. One speaker differentiated control, elimination, and eradication, and observed,

Eradication of a disease as a final target of communicable disease control is not a new idea, especially in veterinary public health. No epidemiologist opposes eradication as a principle. There is practical value, however, in recognizing eradication for what it is—a hope, a laudable ambition, a goal to which to aspire but which, for even the first infectious disease of man, lies a long way ahead.[12]

However, leaving questions of strategy aside, both the 1968 report on smallpox eradication of the WHO Scientific Group and the 1977 report by the WHO Expert Committee on Smallpox Eradication considered the global eradication of smallpox to be "well within the bounds of possibility."[13]

In outlining the planning and execution of mass vaccination program, the WHO Scientific Group in 1968 observed that

> The objective of a mass vaccination programme is the successful vaccination of the entire population of an area in the briefest possible time and in co-ordination with similar programmes in adjacent areas. . . . In general, when 80 percent of each village, social, sex and age group are immunized, smallpox transmission should cease. In densely populated areas, however, higher proportions may be required.[14]

As we have seen, there was ample reason for WHO—as well as the Pan American Health Organization (PAHO) in the Americas and the U.S. Agency for International Development (AID) and the U.S. Communicable Disease Center (CDC) in West Africa—to define the problem, in the early stages, as a problem of mass vaccination.

In retrospect, however, that definition of the problem may be seen as a classical case of confusion of means and objectives or ends. The effect of that confusion on the world wide eradication campaign was profound, and for that reason an examination of the process of organizational learning that occurred is vitally important. *Indeed, that process, more than any other element in the campaign, is the key explanatory factor of the ultimate success of the program.*

Not infrequently, individuals and organizations reconstruct events, history, and the development of strategies *post facto*, and in retrospect infuse more order, system, and logic into such processes than actually existed. The process by which the smallpox eradication campaign defined the problem, learned organizationally, and altered strategy is no exception. This was recognized implicitly by the director of the WHO campaign some time after the shift of strategy from mass vaccination to surveillance and containment had occurred:

> In the development of the global program, it thus seemed more logical to reconsider the strategy in terms of the actual objective, "eradication of smallpox," and to determine how best to interrupt completely transmission

of the disease rather than to focus attention solely on methods to vaccinate all the people.[15]

It is clear, in hindsight, that an imprecise definition of the problem— that is, defining the problem as *mass vaccination* rather than *eradication*— created a serious obstacle in terms of change of strategy. Intellectually and organizationally, early definitions of problems often cause long-lasting effects on subsequent thought processes and organizational action.

"Organizational learning," of course, is a shorthand concept. Obviously, organizations do not learn; members of organizations can and do (sometimes) learn. Organizational learning occurs within a framework (typically based upon initial problem definition) provided by organizational structures, their complex relationships, rules, and communication networks. These aspects also serve to condition, facilitate, restrict, and sometimes prevent the learning and adaptation process.

For these reasons, organizational structures, including control devices, rules, feedback mechanisms, and evaluation techniques, are important for understanding of response, innovation, and change. How did the smallpox eradication organization communicate internally and externally in the process of controlling programs? What evaluation systems operated to insure timely and effective interpretation of field results? These and similar questions are important for analysis of the learning and adaptation that occurred as the global eradication campaign progressed after 1966.

Repeated references exist in the literature of epidemiology about the concept of surveillance and epidemiologic control and its importance. For example, the Royal Commission on Vaccination in 1896 advocated epidemiologic control methods when it became clear that mass vaccination methods were not eliminating smallpox in England. The commission pointed out the need for a "complete system of notification."[16]

Dixon's classic text on smallpox[17] suggested that more study be given to smallpox foci as a means of eliminating smallpox by vaccinating a much smaller proportion of the population. He dismissed the notion that smallpox eradication could be achieved by vaccinating 80 percent of the population within four or five years. However, Dixon's concern was more on outbreak control than on broad strategy.[18]

Other fragmentary approaches to surveillance and containment developed slowly and were accepted slowly. The approach was used mainly in non-endemic countries trying to eliminate importations of smallpox.[19] In the history of smallpox control in the United States, no clear national strategy is evident. What really happened was that local jurisdictions reacted to outbreaks *with their own form of surveillance-containment.*

These local containment actions took various forms. An outbreak of smallpox in Seattle and King County, Washington, in 1946 originated from a soldier returning from Kyushu, Japan. The result was 51 cases, of which 16 (31.6 percent) were fatal. The outbreak stimulated a mass vaccination program in which some 350,000 people out of a population of 475,000 were vaccinated in an emergency effort. Similar vaccination campaigns were carried out in San Francisco and other coastal cities, including Vancouver and Victoria in British Columbia.[20]

Similar, but more extensive steps were taken as a result of an outbreak of smallpox in New York City in 1947. The outbreak originated from a merchant who came to New York by bus from Mexico City, and led to 12 cases, of whom two died. As soon as smallpox was suspected, all employees and patients of the hospital where the merchant entered were vaccinated. An emergency vaccination program was started quickly and within less than a month more than 6,350,000 people were vaccinated, over 5 million of them in less than two weeks. The Commissioner of Health of New York City, who described the outbreak, noted that

had vaccination not been carried out on such a large scale, there very likely would have been thousands of cases and hundreds of deaths. . . . Universal vaccination is the only safeguard. . . . Just as soon as a case of smallpox is suspected in a community, every effort must be made to have everyone vaccinated without delay.[21]

An outbreak of smallpox in the lower Rio Grande Valley of Texas in 1949 was controlled by means of a localized mass vaccination campaign. Some 106,000 persons were vaccinated in Hidalgo County, 103,000 in Cameron County, and 30,000 in Starr County. One person died as a result of the outbreak.[22]

What Seattle, New York City, and Texas were practicing, in effect, was a form of surveillance-containment, albeit on a broader scale than might have been essential. This approach was typical of efforts in non-endemic countries to control isolated outbreaks of smallpox. An extreme example of over-reaction may be seen in the 1972 Yugoslavia situation, which is discussed in more detail below. However, as William Foege pointed out, "science needs more than one example or lesson before it is willing to try a new approach."[23] Good epidemiology, with the benefit of hindsight and experience, might have indicated the need to vaccinate less than 6 million people in the New York City outbreak. But epidemiologists must be sensitive to political factors as well as medical ones. The political pressure, driven by no small amount of terror over the prospect of a smallpox epidemic, was compelling.

The international smallpox eradication campaign is a story of increasing sophistication as the program progressed. There was constant refinement

.in every phase as the attack continued. In West Africa, where the goal was mass vaccination, the initial campaign approach was relatively crude.

In Nigeria, where the new strategy of surveillance-containment was used initially (out of necessity), the first outbreak after that point disappeared so quickly that it seemed like a fluke. However, the field team began to investigate patterns of migration, seasonal variation, and similar factors. Patterns showed importation from the north, gradually drifting south. Accordingly, attention was put where the problem was worst. These data were presented by William Foege at a meeting in Accra in July 1967.[24]

Several factors led to the revised strategy in West Africa: vaccine did not arrive in Nigeria by Christmas 1966 as scheduled; thus selective vaccination was required. An outbreak occurred in Abekaliki; 30 cases developed despite previous vaccination coverage of some 93 percent of the population. A series of maps drawn by Foege by seasons showed a clear pattern of cases. Since one chain of transmission could lead to 75 cases, it made sense to start an attack at the low point. It became obvious that smallpox does not move rapidly—further support of Mack's findings in West Pakistan regarding the fragility of transmission.[25] As the campaign proceeded, field observations demonstrated clearly that smallpox is not one of the more contagious diseases.[26]

Foege argued later that the use of surveillance and containment techniques in smallpox endemic countries

> is a logical extension if endemic countries are viewed as non-endemic areas with "islands" of endemicity, each equivalent to an importation. Removal of the islands is reasonable at any time, but particularly crucial at the seasonal trough period when the fewest islands exist.[27]

Foege pointed out, from his own experience, that (1) high levels of vaccination were not clearly a condition of eradication, and (2) a high level of vaccination was not really needed once smallpox was under basic control.[28]

However, at the time of the Accra meeting in 1967 when the new strategy was broached initially, Foege was not fully sold. Only slowly did realization build up about how compelling the new strategy was.[29]

The new approach, which was identified at the time as *eradication escalation,* or E^2, had several components:

1. Surveillance. (a) *Passive surveillance* used the regular disease-reporting system to determine where control teams should work. This meant waiting for reports. (b) *Active surveillance* attempted to find cases not reported through the regular system. The search employed newspapers, radio, and letters, and cooperated with other government personnel such

as teachers, rural mail carriers, agricultural personnel, village and area chiefs, and volunteer agencies such as missions. Sometimes, house-to-house searches sought out cases and vaccinated persons.

2. Outbreak Investigation. Reported cases were investigated promptly, the extent of the outbreak delineated, and target areas defined. Events which produced the outbreak were established. The teams attempted to trace the chain of infection and collected laboratory specimens to verify the diagnosis.

3. Outbreak Control. The object was "to vaccinate a geographically or sociologically contiguous 'area' around each patient," the extent determined by the investigation. This type of outbreak control was "intermediate between selective vaccination of close personal contacts (practiced to control imported smallpox in many non-endemic countries) and the indiscriminate mass vaccination campaigns. . . ."

4. Communications. Weekly telegraphic reports went to the Smallpox Eradication Unit at CDC and to its regional office in Lagos. Data were circulated in a weekly report and distributed to health officials of the countries involved.[30]

Application of the new strategy began to produce results very quickly. A steady improvement in the percentage of outbreaks investigated occurred in 1968–1969 and all reported outbreaks were investigated in 1969.[31] Tables 4.1 and 4.2 clearly indicate the effects of the new approach. Active surveillance activities resulted in a great increase in the percentage of total cases detected through surveillance. This rose from five percent in the first half of 1968 to between 57 and 67 percent in the period October 1968 to January 1969. Monthly reports for West Africa for 1968 and 1969 were consistently below the corresponding mean for 1960–1967 (except for September 1968, which reflected intensified surveillance). A continued decline in 1969 reached zero in November 1970. In Sierra Leone (with the world's highest rate in 1968), only 66 percent of the population had been vaccinated by May 1969, when smallpox disappeared. In Mali, only 51 percent had been vaccinated.[32] In general, the attack on smallpox foci prevented the expected seasonal increase in 1969 and interrupted transmission throughout West and Central Africa.[33]

In another respect, the 1967 meeting in Accra appears to have had a galvanizing effect on those persons present. According to one participant, the meeting "put a chill down your backbone," and he came to believe *then* that smallpox eradication was a real possibility.[34]

Of course, the new strategy of surveillance-containment was not developed fully in the initial application in West Africa. As one participant observed, the strategy "changed fifteen times." In 1969, a WHO paper outlined the purpose of surveillance-containment as follows:

TABLE 4.1 Number of Reported Smallpox Outbreaks and Percentage Investigated,
January 1968-January 1969*

Time Period	No. of Reported Outbreaks	No. Investigated	% Investigated
January-June 1968† (Monthly Average)	109 (18)	86 (14)	78.7
July-September 1968 (Monthly Average)	91 (30)	77 (26)	84.6
October-December 1968 (Monthly Average)	71 (24)	69 (23)	97.2
January 1969	28	28	100.0

* Dahomey, Ghana, Guinea, Mali, Niger, Northern States Nigeria, Sierra Leone, Togo, and Upper Volta
† Incomplete for Northern States Nigeria

Source: W.H. Foege, J.D. Millar, and J. M. Lane, "Selective Epidemiologic Control in Smallpox Eradication," 94 *American Journal of Epidemiology* (October 1971), p. 314.

- to investigate every suspect case of smallpox notified through conventional reporting channels or through other sources such as malaria personnel, news media, etc.
- to determine the source of infection and to trace the chain of transmission
- to contain the outbreak through:
  —isolation of cases at home or in hospital
  —vaccination of household contacts
  —vaccination of other residents in the area and special groups at risk such as those in schools and hospitals.[35]

In promoting the concept of surveillance-containment, the WHO smallpox eradication program director, D. A. Henderson, observed,

While total vaccination of the entire population is a worthy objective and, if successful, would assure eradication of smallpox, such coverage is logistically and practically impossible. In fact, as efforts are made to increase vaccination coverage beyond 80 percent to 85 percent, the costs and difficulties increase logarithmically while immunity levels increase only arithmetically. Even with 90 percent of the population vaccinated, smallpox transmission may still persist.[36]

TABLE 4.2 Smallpox Reports Received Through Official Reporting Systems and by Active
Surveillance in Selected Countries* of West and Central Africa, January 1968-January 1969

Time Period	Cases Reported Through Official Reporting	Cases Discovered Through Active Surveillance	Total Cases	% Detected Through Active Surveillance
January-June 1968	3865	195	4060	4.8
(Monthly Average)	(644)	(33)	(677)	
July-September 1968	612	216	828	26.1
(Monthly Average	(204)	(72)	(276)	
October 1968	88	177	265	66.8
November 1968	69	146	215	67.9
December 1968	60	80	140	57.2
January 1969	54	76	130	58.4

* Dahomey, Ghana, Guinea, Mali, Niger, Northern States Nigeria, Sierra Leone, Togo, and Upper Volta
† Incomplete for Northern States Nigeria

Source: W.H. Foege, J.D. Millar, and J. M. Lane, "Selective Epidemiologic Control in Smallpox Eradication," 94
American Journal of Epidemiology (October 1971), p. 314.

It would be misleading to suggest that the new strategy of surveillance-
containment was accepted immediately and completely—by the field, by
WHO and CDC, or by the host countries themselves. When Foege
presented his thinking at the 1968 Lagos meeting, the initial reaction
was "sort of skeptical." Foege even earlier had raised the idea at CDC
with Millar—why not hit smallpox at a low point? Millar agreed the
idea was novel and suggested that it be tried. But he did not accept the
idea of dropping mass vaccination completely; rather, surveillance-containment should be tried along with it. Donald Hopkins clearly thought
surveillance-containment was a workable concept and used it successfully
with dramatic results in Sierra Leone in 1968. (The eradication campaign
continued to complete the program in West Africa and overall vaccination
coverage was quite high, largely because the CDC Participating Agency
Service Agreement (PASD) with AID called for certain levels of performance regarding coverage.)[37] The use of the new strategy of eradication
escalation (that came to be known as surveillance-containment) did not

TABLE 4.3 Comparison of Number of Smallpox Vaccinations,
Fourth Quarter 1967 and Fourth Quarter 1968

	No. Vaccinations Performed		
	Fourth Quarter 1967	Fourth Quarter 1968	% Increase
Countries Participating in Eradication Escalation Activities*	4,546,424	6,092,684	34
Other West African Countries	2,137,504	2,287,581	7
Total	6,683,928	8,380,265	25

* Minus Sierra Leone. Sierra Lione did not begin its vaccination campaign until 1968.

Source: W.H. Foege, J.D. Millar, and J. M. Lane, "Selective Epidemiologic Control in Smallpox Eradication," 94 *American Journal of Epidemiology* (October 1971), p. 314.

signify any slackening in the pace of vaccinations. Table 4.3 clearly shows substantial increases between 1967 and 1968.

After the regional meeting in Abidjan in May 1968, a follow-up letter from Millar asked the country directors to try the new strategy and goals were set for every level of jurisdiction.[38]

The responses of host countries to the surveillance-containment strategy varied considerably. For example, in Brazil, as in most places, the dominant strategy was mass vaccination and that approach was deeply ingrained in local health officials. But surveillance-containment was adopted in 1969, shortly after its adoption in Nigeria, and used mainly in Bahia, Minas Gerais, Paraná, and Rio Grande do Sul. The campaign was completed in 1969, having vaccinated 85–90 percent of the people.[39] In areas such as Gabon, where the French *Service des Grandes Enfermies* had operated very effectively since the end of the Second World War, little change occurred in the basic strategy of mass vaccination.

Writing about the experience of the West African campaign, an operations officer in the program referred to surveillance-containment (then called "eradication escalation") almost as if it were simply a special refinement in what would continue to be principally a mass vaccination program:

When properly conducted in association with mass vaccination activities, there need be no significant decrease in the total vaccinations administered, although the programme has shown that in some cases some decrease in effective supervision may occur. . . . It is already apparent that mass vaccination techniques must continue as the most important part of maintenance activities.[40]

According to one participant, Donald Millar (from CDC) acted with "considerable grace" in accepting the implication of surveillance-containment, which represented a radical shift of policy and strategy for CDC and the eradication campaign.[41]

Even in Nigeria, where Foege conceived the strategy of surveillance-containment, the concept was not adopted quickly or totally. In selling the idea, Foege emphasized that surveillance-containment was an addition to a mass vaccination strategy. Foege observed to me that he did not have the courage to fully junk mass vaccination.[42] In Upper Volta, however, French health officials did not change their strategy at all.[43] In traditional Moslem areas, mass vaccination did the job well because leaders could assemble people effectively in large groups.[44] Many local officials, however, were afraid that mass vaccination might be compromised by the new strategy and were reluctant to change. As a general rule, though, surveillance-containment was presented not on an "either-or" basis, but as a "fire-fighting" tactic to be used whenever possible.[45] Many governments liked mass vaccination because it was a visible, relatively cheap way to demonstrate that they were doing something.[46]

The Yugoslavia epidemic of 1972 offers a good example of the unwillingness of governments to trust a relatively new, untested strategy such as surveillance-containment. The outbreak in February 1972 was the first one in over 40 years (the last recorded case of smallpox in Yugoslavia had occurred in 1930), and originated from a Moslem pilgrim infected in Iraq. The outbreak followed a relaxation of routine vaccine requirements, even among hospital staff.

After the diagnosis of suspected cases in the province of Kosovo, 300 kilometers south of Belgrade, was confirmed by the Belgrade Institute of Immunology and Virology, containment measures were put into effect and a widespread vaccination program was started. News of the smallpox outbreak, unfortunately, caused turmoil in the country. The disease was carried to Belgrade by a patient who was diagnosed incorrectly and 37 cases resulted. In a period of four days, 1,200,000 people were vaccinated in some 2,500 vaccination posts manned 24 hours a day. On 24 March, the Yugoslav government decided to vaccinate the entire population. With WHO aid and donations from thirteen nations, more than 15 million doses of vaccine were contributed. The last known case occurred on 10 April 1972. During the epidemic, 175 people contracted smallpox and 35 patients died from the infection.

It is quite certain that careful application of the surveillance-containment strategy in Yugoslavia would have controlled the spread of smallpox in short order. But public outcry and the concern of the government led to probably unnecessary use of mass vaccination. Similar reactions occurred in other countries before surveillance-containment was accepted fully.[47] (The New York City outbreak in 1947 is a typical case, though before use of the new strategy.)

As is often the case with major new approaches, eventually a certain amount of "jockeying" developed over "authorship" or "ownership" of the surveillance-containment strategy. In the early period, there was no pressing need to convince leaders about the new strategy, because CDC was really in control and CDC teams, for the most part, shifted fairly readily to surveillance-containment and new reporting systems. No clearance was obtained from WHO for the shift, though CDC was willing and supportive.[48] The consensus appears to be, however, that gaining acceptance was more a problem in some countries than in WHO.[49] Indeed, surveillance-containment was greeted with some relief in WHO headquarters because it promised a more concentrated strategy.[50] It is apparently true that WHO did not push the concept energetically until the Asian campaign began in earnest. In part, this was due to the fact that, for most purposes, CDC managed the West African campaign. Further, WHO headquarters was involved deeply in its efforts to insure availability of dependable, high-quality vaccine, as well as coordinating broader international support of the worldwide campaign. Most observers agree, nevertheless, that WHO staff appreciated the data and results from West Africa—the new surveillance-containment strategy had proved itself.[51] It was suggested by two participants, however, that surveillance-containment is a "land mine" and that jealousy in WHO about "authorship" is probably worse today than at the time of adoption of the new strategy.[52]

Undoubtedly, much of the time lag in adopting surveillance-containment was "political time"—time to sell the idea. Inertia and traditional modes delayed adoption as people slowly changed their thinking. Indeed, it has been argued that the strategy of mass vaccination set up the possibility for surveillance-containment to work. The Nigeria team considered it good management to do mass vaccination to reduce the number of foci to manageable levels. A series of sweeps of mass vaccination were conducted, then surveillance- containment was used, then periodic re-vaccination campaigns were used to cover newborn children and similar groups. Of course, there was a substantial investment in the mass vaccination approach—salaries, jobs, etc.—and surveillance-containment could be interpreted as criticism of the old ways.[53]

Some of this concern over the origins of surveillance-containment apparently stems from a legitimate interest in understanding the history of the evolution of the E² campaign. Thus, a letter dated 18 August 1976 from D. A. Henderson to Stanley Foster of CDC raised questions about the origins of surveillance-containment, reading, in part:

> Surprisingly, in all the documents I have read of that time [1967–1968], no mention is made of the significance of the early Eastern Nigerian experience, including a report from Bill [Foege] dated March 1967. I'm now beginning to wonder if the seed of the intensified campaign may not have germinated from an entirely different source with that experience being employed later in illustration.[54]

The letter from Henderson enclosed a short paper (written in 1968 by Foster?) which proposed an attack campaign based on analysis of seasonal incidence of smallpox in Nigeria. A series of maps compared the number of cases in the different regions of Nigeria during the "high" period (early March through May) and the "low" period (mid-August through early November). A remarkable difference was obvious; the maps clearly indicated that, in a non-epidemic year, the period of August through October was the period of lowest transmission. The likelihood of eradicating smallpox was highest when transmission was lowest and a much smaller effort would be required. When I raised this matter with Foege, saying that the letter appeared to suggest a problem over "authorship" of E², he agreed but indicated he'd rather not discuss it further. He did go on to say that the question of origin had been sort of a "burr under the saddle" of some people in WHO who were bothered that WHO did not think up the strategy first.[55] Foege again reiterated his earlier observation that surveillance-containment was not really new.

At several points in the worldwide eradication campaign, timing was of absolutely crucial importance. D. A. Henderson observed that there were probably fifty instances where the whole campaign literally "hung by a thread."[56] Timing was critical in the early phases of the use of surveillance-containment. Foege noted that the Biafran civil war disrupted the smallpox campaign so that it was not certain that smallpox was in fact eradicated when Foege left to return to CDC. According to one source, Foege came to a tentative conclusion regarding eradication escalation when he realized in Biafra that total vaccination was impossible because of local conditions.[57] But by 1968, he was convinced that surveillance-containment would work. If the northern Nigerian campaign had been delayed for just two months, the war would have disrupted it totally and the new strategy might never have received a fair test. Considerably later, in 1972, at a meeting of health officials from Southeast Asian countries, several leaders were ready to concede defeat on the ten-year goal of eradication before Foege arose to defend surveillance-containment and convinced them that the strategy could work in India and Bangladesh.[58]

Brilliant describes how, in India, a disastrous epidemic was turned into a positive lesson about the workability of the surveillance-containment strategy. In December 1970, a major outbreak occurred in the Gulbarga district in Karmataka (in southwestern India), and continued until April 1972. The initial outbreak had been concealed by medical officers in the Primary Health Centers, "perhaps due to fear of reprimand, which was a common response to such reports." The epidemic finally got Delhi's attention, however, and all available health personnel were mobilized for a house-to-house search of the area. Within weeks, smallpox was eliminated from the district. The operation in Gulbarga was India's first real success with surveillance-containment, and coming at the same time as the Indonesian victory, the experience was highly persuasive. It proved that the new strategy could work in even the most densely populated country.[59]

Evidence about the effectiveness of surveillance-containment accumulated rapidly. Koswara, taking West Java as an example, demonstrated that surveillance-containment brought smallpox under control in a short period while on the contrary, routine vaccinations and mass vaccination campaigns had little effect in interrupting smallpox transmission.[60]

Henderson, in attempting to promote acceptance of the strategy of surveillance-containment, lamented that

all have not yet fully appreciated the concept that there is no such thing as a single case of smallpox or a small outbreak which develops spontaneously without relationship to other cases or other outbreaks. . . . Subclinical infections play *no* role in transmission of smallpox. In this respect, smallpox is almost unique among the infectious diseases. When one case is detected, it is a certainty that this person acquired the disease from someone else with overt, clinical disease. It is vital that this person be identified and containment measures taken and that the source of infection of the previous case be investigated and so on. . . . in the great majority of cases, the source of infection can be traced back over many generations.[61]

In retrospect, considering the West Africa experience, Foege observed:

Intelligent use of vaccination based on knowledge of where the disease is and when, where, and to whom the disease is likely to spread is more economical in time, vaccine, and personnel than blind mass vaccination. Mass vaccination campaigns should continue in endemic areas, but we consider the use of surveillance, investigation, and selective epidemiologic control techniques to be of equal and, under certain circumstances, of even greater importance than systematic mass vaccination activities.[62]

By the time the India and Bangladesh campaigns were fully underway, surveillance-containment had replaced mass vaccination entirely and there was no further argument that mass vaccination should continue in endemic areas. Surveillance began in East Africa almost from the start, with "ring vaccination" and detection.[63] However, the campaigns in Uganda, Kenya, Ethiopia, and the Ogaden in 1977 were so intensive as to be almost mass vaccination, the purpose being to create an "immune belt."[64]

Development and Refinement of Surveillance and Containment

In retrospectively examining the development of the surveillance-containment strategy, Henderson observes that this approach was emphasized less initially,

> because it was believed that it would first be necessary to reduce smallpox incidence to less that five cases per 100,000 population before the surveillance-containment activities could be effective. It was hoped that systematic vaccination programs designed to reach 80 percent of the population would achieve a reduction in incidence to this level. While such vaccination programs were in progress, sufficient time would be provided for a surveillance system to develop.[65]

My reading of the record does not indicate that any clear and logical, deliberate plan of this sort existed. It *is* entirely clear that surveillance procedures went through a long period of development to fit the particular environments and that surveillance-containment was not a straightforward step from mass vaccination.[66] But it is not at all clear that a surveillance-containment strategy even of the sort envisioned by Foege in Nigeria (which was relatively rudimentary) was *planned* or even envisioned by WHO.[67] However, in 1967 a joint assessment team of Indian and WHO experts, examining the eradication situation in India, declared,

> Mass vaccination alone does not constitute a smallpox eradication programme. Rather the function of mass vaccination is to reduce the incidence of the disease to a sufficiently low level to make it possible for other measures—case detection and containment of outbreaks—to eliminate the remaining endemic foci.[68]

Surveillance means many things. Langmuir defines the concept as follows:

Surveillance, when applied to a disease, means the continued watchfulness over the distribution and trends of incidence through the systematic collection, consolidation and evaluation of morbidity and mortality reports and other relevant data. Intrinsic in the concept is the regular dissemination of the basic data and interpretations to all who have contributed and to all others who need to know.[69]

As Henderson emphasized,

The objective of the surveillance component of the programme quite simply is to investigate every case of smallpox, to trace its source and to take containment action. . . . The moral, quite simply, whether for endemic or non-endemic countries, is that surveillance and immediate containment of smallpox outbreaks is the key to maintaining or achieving a smallpox-free status. This task is considerably simplified if one has a highly immune population and so the need for continuing vaccination programs. Vaccination alone is not likely, however, to result in a smallpox-free status.[70]

Surveillance-containment had been used for years in many forms. In the United Kingdom, for example, mass vaccination was never accepted. In east Africa, facilities would not support mass vaccination, so surveillance was started in Kenya in 1966. A full system of surveillance, however, could not work because of lack of people and funds. Active surveillance, detection, and containment started in Nigeria with Foege. As the strategy evolved in Asia it was more selective, aimed at certain groups. The first full surveillance system began in India, in 1973, when some 200 experts started a very active program of search, detection, outbreak investigation, and full mobilization.[71]

The characteristics of smallpox itself facilitated success of surveillance-containment. The virus is not transmitted until a rash develops, so spread can be reduced by early isolation. Vaccination offers virtually complete protection within 10–12 days. There is an incubation period of two weeks between generation of cases and usually the patient infects no more than two to five additional persons. So prompt action using isolation and vaccination of actual or potential contacts rapidly stops further transmission. Identification of the source of infection is relatively easy because transmission usually requires face to face contact—the chain of transmission can be readily identified and outbreaks detected.[72]

As the campaign matured and better data were available on the characteristics of people who contracted smallpox, vaccination was focused increasingly on high-risk groups:

- More than 85 percent of cases occur among those who have never been vaccinated.

- More than 80 percent occur among children under 15 years of age.
- A disproportionate number occur and persist in immigrant groups in urban slum areas (these serve to introduce smallpox into rural areas).
- The "role of the hospital as one of the most dangerous and common places for dissemination of infection was recognized," so that persons entering an infectious hospital for any reason should be vaccinated.[73]

Whatever might be said about the reception in WHO of the new strategy of surveillance-containment immediately after its adoption in West Africa, there can be no doubt of D. A. Henderson's vigorous promotion of the approach once its effectiveness had been proven clearly. His comments at an interregional seminar in New Delhi (in 1970) are typical:

> I do not mean to belabour unduly the importance of reporting and surveillance but we must bear in mind that *unless an effective reporting and surveillance programme is developed, there is no prospect whatsoever for a successful eradication programme.*[74]

Henderson clearly recognized that the surveillance component was the chief difference between the 1966 campaign and previous eradication efforts. Experience showed that the combination of a good reporting system and vigorous investigation and containment of every outbreak resulted in interruption of smallpox transmission in two years or less in every country where this had been done. However, by the time the WHO Expert Committee on Smallpox Eradication issued its second report (1972), the smallpox eradication program had accumulated five years of experience, and as a result, references to mass vaccination virtually disappeared in the 1972 report. The second report reflected the lessons learned since 1968, especially from the further development of the surveillance-containment strategy. The Committee noted: "In the past, eradication programmes consisted almost solely in mass vaccination; the present strategy places greater emphasis on surveillance." The Committee went on to observe:

> In addition to its usefulness in defining high-risk groups, [persons never vaccinated and persons under 15 years old] surveillance has an even more important part to play in interrupting the transmission of smallpox. . . . The remarkable efficacy of surveillance and containment measures may be explained by the epidemiological behavior of smallpox. . . . A person does not usually transmit the disease to more than 2 or 3 additional persons, and transmission generally takes place as a result of face-to-face

contact in the home, hospital, or school. Outbreaks thus develop rather slowly under most circumstances and are mostly confined to geographically limited areas. Containment measures, consisting primarily in intensive vaccination of contacts and their near neighbours, are usually effective in stopping transmission. . . . Surveillance has thus been the keystone of the strategy for smallpox eradication.[75]

The committee thus gave its unqualified support to the surveillance and containment strategy.

Writing in 1972, Henderson clearly recognized the shift from the strategy of mass vaccination to the approach where surveillance-containment was the key element as the most important reason for the program's great achievements between 1967 and 1971.[76]

By 1975, Henderson was describing surveillance as

the most powerful, effective, and underrated tool in communicable disease control. . . . In essence, it represents organically the brain and nervous system in a management process. As we in preventive medicine begin to understand and employ some of the more modern approaches to management, the surveillance mechanism . . . will assume an increasing if not dominant role not only in monitoring disease incidence but in monitoring the operation of the programme as a whole.[77]

In its 1980 report on the campaign, WHO recognizes that eradication campaigns that were based entirely or mainly on the strategy of mass vaccination failed in most countries, although they succeeded in some. The successful mass vaccination campaigns occurred generally where health services were well developed and well managed and where adequate reporting systems and good communications existed. But in other countries, even if mass vaccination reached 80 or even 90 percent of the population, enough susceptibles remained for smallpox transmission to continue. Reaching a higher level of coverage would have been very costly and difficult if not impossible to achieve.[78]

Plan and Strategy Modification

The major strategy change—from mass vaccination to surveillance and containment—was followed by other shifts as field reports were sifted and interpreted. The organization proved itself capable of recognizing the need for change in tactics as experience accumulated and then acting on that need.

For example, field data clearly showed that smallpox cases among adult females were extremely rare. As a result, a program to vaccinate women isolated by *purdah* was dropped. Data from Africa and South America indicated that over 95 percent of all cases occurred among people who had never been vaccinated. So emphasis was shifted to primary vaccination. This lesson could have been learned much earlier. In this respect, Brilliant notes a "fatal error" in the Indian National Smallpox Eradication Program in the 1960s, where equal emphasis was given to both revaccination and primary vaccination, largely because the target for revaccination were easily accessible sectors such as school children and industrial workers.[79] Intensive surveillance and reporting also indicated that smallpox could be eliminated frequently with less than half the population vaccinated.[80] It is probably accurate to say, however, that once surveillance-containment was formulated and tested successfully, WHO consistently applied the new strategy (of course, refining it steadily) throughout the campaign.[81] Foege observed that new systems were added constantly to the basic strategy and it took some 18 months to really refine and master the system.[82] The epidemiologic pattern was described and reanalyzed periodically to develop positive control measures and to change approaches and tactics according to changes in the epidemiologic situation.

When Foege got to India in 1973, the strategy was (1) find cases and (2) contain the outbreaks. In October 1973, a village-by-village search in Uttar Pradesh and Bihar discovered 10,000 new cases. The capacity to contain was almost overwhelmed. The basic approach shifted to a house-by-house search, then market surveillance, catching people as they entered or left the market. Houses were marked after each search. Once a refinement became a matter of habit or routine, attention could be put on new approaches. Smallpox disappeared in some 19 months before the strategy was ever fully worked out.[83] One consultant described the Indian campaign as an "unrelenting search for perfection."[84]

Evolution of Strategy: Bangladesh

An example of a gradual shift of strategy, based upon constant organizational learning, may be seen in the Bangladesh campaign. As in other countries, campaign strategy in Bangladesh evolved gradually from mass vaccination to surveillance-containment. Figure 4.2 shows the evolution of the containment strategy. The goal of the scheme which was started in 1961 was mass vaccination of the entire population by 1963. The government in 1965 acknowledged that, in spite of 75 million vaccinations during the three years 1961, 1962, and 1963, smallpox continued. Although a radical change in emphasis toward case detection and outbreak containment was proposed at the Dacca conference in October 1969, the program strategy set forth in December 1969 still emphasized mass vaccination. But the need for concurrent assessment was recognized. Passive reporting eventually was supplemented by three

FIGURE 4.2 Evolution of the Containment Strategy, 1972-1975

Year	Problems Identified	Solution Introduced
1972-1973	Need for containment of outbreaks recognised	Isolation of patients attempted. Vaccination of available residents of nearest 30 houses
	Transmission continuing among those absent during the day	One late evening or early morning vaccination round in each infected village
1974	Increased smallpox incidence Frequent containment failures Insufficient liaison with village community	GHA* joined by one EFW** to form a team resident in infected village for at least 10 days. Detailed vaccination programmes using JL maps Clearly defined roles Improved supervision and reporting
1975	Continued containment failures	Additional manpower including up to 12 EFWs for vaccination and surveillance Extension of containment area
	Difficulty in maintaining isolation of patients	Initally four, later six EFWs appointed as House Guards
	Patients leaving isolation for marketing or to earn income	Food provided to patients and families where necessary
	Lack of continuous supervision	Outbreak Supervisor, and later Resident Supervisors for each Zone, appointed
	Need for measurement of containment efficiency	Quantitive objective: no new cases to occur 15 or more days after detection of outbreak.
	House missed during containment activities	Maps of containment area drawn
	Spread via unvaccinated persons and patients' relatives	Containment Books listing all residents and visitors within a half-mile radius of the infected house, and all patients' relatives
	Undetected spread from second generation cases	Containment period extended to end six weeks or more after onset of last case

* GHA = Government Health Assistant
** EFW = Emergency Field Worker

Source: WHO. The Eradication of Smallpox from Bangladesh, p. 53.

systems of surveillance—market surveillance, infected village surveillance, and house-to-house surveillance. Markets proved to be a fruitful source of reports because at least one person from every family visited a market once or twice weekly. Market patterns, in terms of days of operation and location, were found to be remarkably consistent over a period of many decades. This facilitated the preparation of plans for surveillance and containment visits. The shift to infected village surveillance was based on the fact that the containment action to be taken was independent of the number of cases found, because the entire village would be vaccinated, in any case. The resurgence of smallpox in Bangladesh after the severe floods of 1974 (the worst in 20 years) led to intensification of the campaign through house-to-house surveillance, including eventually search for all cases of rash and fever. The intensified search even caused a sense of competition to develop among health workers. Some 87 percent of about 15 million houses in the country were visited ultimately.

Surveillance workers in Bangladesh learned to avoid the specific Bengali term for smallpox when searching. Using the more general term for "pox," which included a variety of skin diseases, increased the probability that smallpox would be reported. It was not unusual to have both chickenpox and smallpox in the same village at the same time.[85]

Public recognition of health workers and rewards for reporting outbreaks helped change the outlook of health staff. Then in 1975, house-to-house searches, preceded by definite "presearch" programs by house number and "presearch" meetings at the *thana* level greatly improved search effectiveness. Feedback at the next "presearch" meeting in terms of recognition or discipline helped improve search coverage dramatically. A surveillance newsletter with up-to-date reports was distributed regularly.[86]

Clear plans for containing outbreaks were included in the 1974 Emergency Plan in Bangladesh. Two family welfare workers and one locally-recruited emergency field worker were posted to each infected village for ten days to carry out 100 percent vaccination within an 800-meter radius of the infected house and search within a 3-kilometer radius. Thus their work could be checked and corrective steps taken if needed.[87]

The experience in Bangladesh exemplifies the type of organizational learning that characterized the global campaign. All the changes in surveillance and containment strategies were the product of careful field testing, problem identification, and failure analysis. And—extremely important—every action kept foremost the ultimate objective: *the control of every single case of smallpox.*[88]

Evolution of Strategy: Nepal

As the smallpox eradication campaign accrued experience, procedures essentially stabilized, having become steadily more refined. The evolution of strategy in Nepal provides an instructive example of how strategy evolved in the campaign generally.[89]

As in a number of other countries, the smallpox eradication program in Nepal was a special project, a vertical program in the sense that funding and staffing were independent of other programs of the Department of Health Services. Further, all smallpox eradication work was carried out by personnel of the campaign, who had that as their sole responsibility. The regular basic health service officers had no responsibility for smallpox eradication except for reporting of cases.[90]

A pilot smallpox program started in 1962 with the object of vaccinating 80–90 percent of the population of Kathmandu valley. The intention was to create a "sufficiently high herd immunity" in the densely populated valley, and to include other areas gradually. Freeze-dried vaccine and the multiple-pressure vaccination technique were used from the start. But achievement of the target immunity level was difficult because of administrative problems as well as religious and mundane objections of some sectors.

In 1965 a new agreement was signed between WHO and the government of Nepal. Improvement of the reporting system was a stated objective, along with (1) vaccinating or revaccinating 90 percent of the population of Kathmandu valley, and (2) vaccinating newborn children and immigrants and revaccinating as indicated by circumstances. By 1966 Nepal and WHO were discussing the possibility of eradication rather than controlling smallpox. Three main objectives were set (for all of Nepal):

1. immunization programs for the groups most exposed
2. development of routine early detection, isolation, treatment, and rehabilitation
3. development of an organization for routine and prompt focal preventive measures

In 1967 a definitive plan for a smallpox eradication program was signed. The basic strategy was to cover the entire population, following the classic pattern of preparation, attack, and maintenance phases. Epidemiological surveillance would be initiated as early as possible. Experience in the rest of the world (especially in West Africa) led to a complete change of program strategy in 1971 and adoption of the surveillance-containment system. Reporting and record systems were simplified. The only vaccination record was a simple tally sheet showing the number of primary vaccinations and revaccinations performed. Containment was emphasized in 1971 and entire villages were vaccinated if infected. Tracing of the source of infection became a key part of the strategy. From 1971, regular annual refresher training was given to all supervisory staff. Four national surveillance teams were formed in 1972.

These surveillance teams in Nepal, which were to work under the supervision and guidance of the assessment teams, were intended to supplement the regular surveillance systems of the district. The assessment team prepared advanced tour itineraries, focusing on high-risk areas and visits to schools, tea shops, factories, brick kilns, important weekly markets, malaria offices and health posts, and fairs. The teams showed the recognition card, inquired about smallpox, publicized the 1,000 rupee reward, and collected details on suspect cases.[91] The assessment team assessed the performance of district staff and supervised and guided the surveillance teams. In addition, it carried out pockmark surveys of children under five years of age and all persons in special surveys such as the Tibetan refugee camps, and investigated suspect cases.[92]

Very specific and detailed instructions were worked out for immediate containment measures if a smallpox outbreak occurred after apparent eradication. Every outbreak was to be treated as a health emergency. The entire locality would be enumerated and the source of infection located. Then the locality's people would be vaccinated as quickly as possible, in the following priority:

First, households affected
Second, 50 neighboring households
Third, remaining population in the locality
Fourth, remaining people in the *panchayat* and in a one-mile radius[93]

The "watchguard" system (from Indian experience) was adopted in 1975 to prevent infectious patients from leaving their homes and unvaccinated people from entering. Watchguards (two at a time) were placed at every infected house round the clock, so that at least one guard would be present all the time. They were responsible for preventing the smallpox patients from going out of the house and keeping them isolated, restricting entry of visitors and vaccinating all persons coming to the house, keeping records of all contacts leaving for other areas or of those who might have had contacts before containment, and disposal of scabs and fomites.[94] In March 1975 a reward of 100 rupees was offered for information leading to discovery of previously unknown outbreaks. This reward was increased to 1,000 rupees in July 1975. The last case of smallpox in Nepal occurred in Morang district on 6 April 1975. New operational guidelines were written for the "post-zeropox period" for continued surveillance in the districts, and in 1976, two national assessment teams were formed.

In many respects, the Nepal experience provides a good example of how the WHO smallpox eradication campaign organization learned from the continued experience of earlier strategies and incorporated that learning into the design of effective control strategies.

The Task Environment

The experience of the smallpox eradication campaign, a multinational effort of vast proportion, demonstrated dramatically the necessity for cultural adaptations. The campaign operated in many different countries and cultures so that field personnel had to become adept and ingenious in adapting to local cultures. As much as in any public health program in history, the campaign personnel had to be aware of and incorporate the imperatives of the task environment. Many examples illustrate their flexibility.

Traveling variolators had caused small outbreaks of smallpox as they moved from village to village. When the WHO teams persuaded them to accept supplies of freeze-dried vaccine, variolation was stopped in most areas. In another area, where children were tattooed traditionally as a protection against witchcraft, the scars of smallpox immunization came to be accepted for the same purpose. In a country approaching independence, a respected political leader convinced the people that a vaccination scar was a sign of their independence. In another country, vaccinations were combined with census-taking, political meetings, and alphabet-learning and reading programs to save on transportation and time costs. Village midwives came to serve as advance motivators and helped persuade mothers to bring their children. Smallpox teams awaited nomads at wells and waterholes to increase coverage. Recognition that the majority of the people in Africa listen to radio led to use of well-chosen messages by radio.[95] In India, smallpox was so common that the disease had its own goddess, Shitala Mata, and many people believed that smallpox cases were blessings of the goddess. Overcoming or adapting to such beliefs was a major challenge for the vaccination teams.[96] These and other examples illustrate the determined effort by the Smallpox Eradication Unit to maintain its flexibility, to learn, and to innovate as the campaign progressed.

There was considerable cultural resistance to smallpox vaccination in many parts of the world. For example, in Dahomey, among neighboring tribes in Togo, and among many Yoruba in Western Nigeria, smallpox was believed to be a supernatural phenomenon or a divine visitation by a deity. The disease was viewed as punishment for wrongdoing, and "the proper corrective measures are ceremonial and sacrificial, not vaccination."[97] The local herbalist or *fetisheur* had responsibility for care of the sick and protection of the village from medical ills. Resistance to vaccination might come from villagers who conceived of smallpox as a social or supernatural stigma or from *fetisheurs* who saw the vaccination as a threat to their standing. Preparatory meetings with village chiefs were found to be effective in increasing turnout and participation. Some chiefs were even resentful if one village was picked first or over another.[98]

Jezek notes how the eradication campaign in India adapted to find more effective means of dealing with local people. For example, women would be used as vaccinators in some areas because men could not enter homes. Workers from lower castes were employed to work with lower caste people. In Somalia, the campaign tried to use tribal workers who would be accepted more readily. There the eradication campaign had to train local people quickly because only some one percent of the staff were health workers. In both campaigns there was little jealousy over status of M.D.s and professional health workers because everyone was too busy.[99]

The campaign in India had to contend with widespread indifference and sometimes hostility to vaccination, especially among people in the rural areas. Frequently children were hidden from vaccinators, epidemiologists were chased out of villages, and there was a common attitude of indifference and apathy towards such public health measures. A similar situation existed in Bangladesh. Stanley Music observes that in the initial stages of developing a coherent containment policy in Bangladesh, an "almost military style attack" on infected villages would be mounted.

> In the hit-and-run excitement of such a campaign, women and children were often pulled out from under beds, from behind doors, from within latrines, etc. People were chased and, when caught, vaccinated. Many misunderstandings arose and tempers often flared in these heated situations. Attempts were made to secure the cooperation and "blessing" of village headmen, thereby putting social pressure on the villagers. . . . None of this action was intended to be malicious in any sense. However, such campaigns did ignore the culture and sensitivities of rural Bangladesh. Quite a lot of ill will and resentment was created in the process. . . . We went from door to door and vaccinated. When they ran, we chased. When they locked their doors, we broke down their doors and vaccinated them.[100]

Some of these attitudes stemmed from the belief of the people that smallpox is a sign of favor from the goddess Shitala Mata. Certain castes took no precautions at all. Empirically-oriented epidemiologists might understand that a person contracts smallpox because of a viral infection, but a follower of traditional medicine saw "physical entities, plus equally real supernatural bodies, plus metaphysical laws of interaction."[101] Traditional medicine "understands illness in terms of an integrated body-mind-spirit." Many Indians "did not feel enthusiasm for the program . . . because [it] did not satisfy a need which they expected medical practice to meet: to explain a personal event in both personal and cosmic terms."[102] Many people believed simply that smallpox could not be prevented, that the goddess' action was inevitable. Even if they believed in a cure, a majority turned to religious ceremonies for it.[103]

> Communication between the program and the public must be honest, and it must flow in both directions. It is essential that program staff be fully knowledgeable about the community's beliefs about disease and its causation. The cultural interpretations of smallpox varied so dramatically every hundred miles that the various traditional views needed to be learned by the Indian as well as the foreign smallpox staff. Other countries and programs may have differing problems, but the way disease is perceived by the community must be understood and respected.[104]

S. H. Hassan, a participant in the Indian campaign, writing about the religious ceremonies in Bihar that were related to the goddess of smallpox, Shitala Maya, observed:

> There are many written stories, songs and beliefs that influence the behaviour patterns of individuals. Many people believe in spirits that can change the natural order of events. It is proved by the fact that all resort to prayer. Thousands, at this very moment, are probably imploring some supposed power to interfere in their behalf. Thousands ask to be protected from evil. With innovation and scientific advancement these concepts grow less intense. Even then they still exist in the memory of the people in the vast rural area. Health workers must remember these facts. A sound health education program is an essential component for any adventure in the sphere of health services.[105]

One participant in India observed,

> It was hard to convince locals that certain things were essential—such as traveling at night and camping in villages. Setting an example helped enormously. Being foreign helped in many cases. Throwing a temper tantrum to make a point was effective and was forgiven because a foreigner did it.[106]

From the Bangladesh campaign, another consultant noted,

> The one supervisory activity that can forestall or eliminate the most personnel problems is the field visit. A simple exhibit of interest in what the employee

is doing and a willingness to share some of his hardships—e.g., walking twenty miles to see a case he's discovered—is so rare in the Bangladesh civil service that its performance works wonders. The more difficult the journey, the most personnel value to be gained.[107]

Another consultant in the Indian campaign sadly reflected,

> Idealism is a product of elite society—you have to be able to afford it. Idealism is rare in less developed countries. One had to be able to put on blinders in order to deal with smallpox. Smallpox workers had to ignore the great mass of other problems.
>
> American notions of order, schedules, etc., were alien. People would always say "yes" to please. It was hard to motivate people. Phony reports were a serious problem. The caste system was still as strong as ever and this sometimes interferred with dealing with higher caste people. Urban people were much more adept at deception and ingratiation. M.D.s were among the worst for trying to "rip off" the smallpox campaign.[108]

In Brazil, health educators were used to prepare towns a week before the eradication teams arrived. These workers talked with mayors, priests, physicians, and sometimes clubs, and generally this advance work assured good cooperation. There were some problems of rumors among less educated people—for example, rumors that the smallpox eradication program was to sterilize people.[109]

The surveillance teams also encountered a number of important differences between urban and rural smallpox surveillance. One participant described Indian village governments as more corrupt and inefficient, but rural people as cooperative and "beautiful." In the cities of Uttar Pradesh, the opposite was true: government health personnel were excellent and cooperative, but urban residents were difficult to work with.[110] Some of the other differences noted by Orenstein between the environments for urban and rural smallpox surveillance are outlined in Figure 4.3.

Other culturally related problems arose in India. In Uttar Pradesh, for example, a group of people with master's degrees were hired by the WHO consultant—against the advice of local health authorities. Severe problems were created by the group over status, the performance of certain kinds of work, etc. All had to be fired in order to avoid charges of discrimination between Hindus and Moslems.[111]

In Bangladesh, in the old system, smallpox cases were reported only reluctantly—this made the superior look bad. Even in the final stages of the campaign, some health workers were unwilling to report, but the reward system helped overcome this.[112] Another participant recalls,

FIGURE 4.3 Difficulties Encountered in Urban vs. Rural Smallpox Surveillance

	Rural	Urban
1. Community	• Distinct • Closeknit Interactions	• Indistinct • Lack of interactions with neighbors
2. Leadership	• Strong local leadership, usually	• Often weak or non-existent • No local or community-level government
3. Transient Population	• Small, usually relatives and wandering craftsman	• Large, including relatives, shoppers, migrants, workers, beggars, tourists
4. Turnover of Population	• Slow	• Rapid, particularly in slum areas
5. Schools	• Usually easily located	• No central listing
6. Geographic Community	• Well-defined, with previously determined populations	• Poorly defined, with poor estimates of population and and houses
7. Staff	• Large, often well-led	• Pitifully small

Source: Walter A. Orenstein (CDC), 8 May 1981.

a pervasive sense of fatalism is the most pungent impression one derives from contact with Bengali public health administration. Accustomed to being presented with huge problems against which he [the Bengali administrator] can mobilize few—if any—resources, he is likely to retreat quickly into the bureaucratic maze of memos and referrals to higher authority whenever challenged.[113]

Incentives

A variety of incentives was employed in various countries to encourage performance, especially in surveillance activities. In countries where the social system or norms of hierarchical organization discouraged accurate reporting of smallpox cases, as in India and Bangladesh in particular, it was necessary to devise means to overcome that problem. In several countries, the reporting of smallpox outbreaks was interpreted by some as a reflection on their performance in routine vaccination. In some cases, reporting cases even resulted in reprimand or discipline. In effect there was a negative incentive to report accurately. Even at the national level, adjustments sometimes were made to statistics to make them "respectable."

Eventually, financial rewards were offered in several countries for the reporting of previously undetected cases. This reward in India finally reached 1,000 rupees by 1974, a very substantial incentive sometimes amounting to several months' wages.[114] At first, health workers were excluded at the government's insistence. Finally, when WHO persisted, health workers were made eligible and some were even encouraged to go over heads of their superiors to report cases.[115] Many people criticized the large amount of money that was paid as bounties to health workers and officials in India, because the people were paid extra to do what they should do routinely anyway.[116] But the system seemed to work. One WHO consultant even gave out toffee candies as an incentive to those who showed a vaccination scar.[117]

Bangladesh introduced a reward of 50 *taka* ($6.00) in August 1974 for reporting a newly detected smallpox outbreak. An unexpected consequence was that initially health workers did not publicize the reward in order to keep the public from claiming it. The solution was to offer a double reward—one for the first person from the public to report a case and another for the first health worker to confirm the outbreak.[118]

In Bangladesh, the surveillance workers, in addition to showing the vivid recognition card and asking villagers if they had seen anyone like the photograph of a child with smallpox eruptions, would also speak of the reward of 50 *takas* for providing a report about smallpox cases. This reward increased, as the incidence of smallpox fell, to 500 *takas* by the end of 1975, an amount which equaled about two months wages for a day laborer. Eventually more than 90 percent of the households in the country knew about the reward.[119]

In some countries, incentive payments were not used. In Guinea, for example, such payments would have been viewed as "anti-revolutionary" and "corruptive." When widespread search began, many lay workers were hired and WHO provided supplemental pay. Eradication teams kept cash to enable quick hires and deals on the spot. Cash was needed for quick flow and rapid decisions.[120]

Incentives to encourage people to cooperate with the program were not always positive or in the form of reward. Eradicators in Indian cities sometimes used what amounted to extortion to get people to take vaccination. People on occasion were threatened with loss of their food ration cards, or with having the names of family members erased if they were not vaccinated. Since the cards were essential for survival, this tactic worked.[121]

The other major organizational device used to encourage faithful and accurate reporting was the separation of the surveillance and containment functions. Initially surveillance and containment activities were performed by the same teams. The results was, in effect, a conflict of interest, given the prevalent social and bureaucratic norms in some countries.

Health workers are expected to demonstrate good results. Like all humans, they tend to find evidence which supports expectations, and to avoid evidence that doesn't. Workers responsible for controlling a disease [the containment function] will tend to understate its incidence [the surveillance function]. The separation of surveillance and control functions proved to be important.[122]

This move, a fairly subtle organizational change, served, in effect, as a form of internal control and assessment.

We turn in the following chapter to consideration of the technological innovations that facilitated the smallpox eradication campaign.

Notes

1. Chris Argyris, "Making the Undiscussable and Its Undiscussability Discussable," 40 *Public Administration Review* (May/June 1980), 206.

2. Carolyn Buie, "The Smallpox Campaign: A Study in Management Flexibility," PASITIM Design Notes, No. 14.(Bloomington: International Development Institute, 1979.)

3. Lawrence B. Brilliant. *The Management of Smallpox Eradication in India.* (Ann Arbor: The University of Michigan Press, 1985), p. 10.

4. WHO Doc. A19/P&B/2, 28 March 1966, p. 107.

5. Smallpox Eradication Program. National Communicable Disease Center. "Summary: Efficacy and Safety of Intradermal Smallpox Vaccination by Jet Injection." August 10, 1967.

6. J. D. Millar, L. Morris, A. Macedo Filho, Th. M. Mack, W. Dyal, and A. A. Medeiros, "The Introduction of Jet Injection Mass Vaccination into the National Smallpox Eradication Program of Brazil." 23 *Trop. geogr. Med.* (1971), 89–101. See also NCDC. *Report to the Pan American Health Organization of Evaluation of Use of Jet Injection in Smallpox Vaccination in Brazil, January 16-March 3, 1965.* (n.d.)

7. Even with this clear policy choice, there was a suggestion that other epidemiologic approaches could be effective. To protect the population against reimportation, the "ring" vaccination method was suggested, with vaccination, isolation, and/or surveillance of contacts and possible contacts. WHO/Smallpox/10, 7 July 1959, p. 2.

8. "Organization of a Smallpox Eradication Service," WHO/Smallpox/10, 7 July 1959, p. 1.

9. "Organization of a Smallpox Eradication Campaign," WHO/Smallpox/ 20, 25 May 1964, p. 1.

10. D. A. Henderson, "Epidemiology in the Global Eradication of Smallpox," 1 *International Journal of Epidemiology* (1972), 27. The report is WHO Technical Report Series No. 283, 1964.

11. "Outline for Plan of Operation for the Global Smallpox Eradication Project," WHO Doc. PA/66, p. 180.

12. K. Raska, "Global Eradication of Smallpox," WHO SE/66.2, p. 2.

13. *Smallpox Eradication,* WHO Technical Report Series No. 393, (Geneva: WHO, 1968), and *WHO Expert Committee on Smallpox Eradication.* Second Report. WHO Technical Report Series No. 493. (Geneva: WHO, 1972).

14. *Smallpox Eradication.* WHO Technical Report Series No. 393 (Geneva: WHO, 1968), p. 34.

15. D. A. Henderson, "Smallpox Surveillance in the Strategy of Global Eradication," WHO/SE/72.8, p. 1.

16. Royal Commission on Vaccination. *A Report* (London: 1896), as quoted by William H. Foege, J. Donald Millar, and J. Michael Lane, "Selected Epidemiologic Control in Smallpox Eradication," 94 *American Journal of Epidemiology* (October 1971), 315.

17. C. W. Dixon, *Smallpox* (London: J & A Churchill, Ltd., 1962), p. 359, as quoted by Foege, Millar, and Lane, *op. cit.*

18. Interview, J. Donald Millar (CDC), 15 May 1981.

19. William H. Foege, *et al.,* "Selected Epidemiologic Control . . . ," 315.

20. Emil E. Palmquist, "The 1946 Smallpox Experience in Seattle," 38 *Canadian Journal of Public Health* (May 1947), 213–218. See also the article, "Control Measures in British Columbia," 318ff, in the same issue.

21. Israel Weinstein, "An Outbreak of Smallpox in New York City," 37 *American Journal of Public Health* (November 1947), 1376–1384.

22. J. V. Irons, Thelma D. Sullivan, E. B. M. Cook, George W. Cox, and R. A. Hale, "Outbreak of Smallpox in the Lower Rio Grande Valley of Texas in 1949." 43 *American Journal of Public Health* (Jan. 1953), 25–29.

23. Interview, William Foege (CDC), 13 May 1981.

24. *Ibid.*

25. Interview, Stanley Foster (CDC), 7 May 1981.

26. William H. Foege, J. Donald Millar, and J. Michael Lane, "Selected Epidemiologic Control in Smallpox Eradication," 94 *American Journal of Epidemiology* (October 1971), 311.

27. William H. Foege, *et al.,* "Selected Epidemiologic control . . . ," 315.

28. Interview, R. C. Hogan (WHO), 6 October 1981.

29. Interview, William Foege (CDC), 13 May 1981.

30. William H. Foege, *et al.,* "Selected Epidemiologic Control . . . ," 312–313.

31. *Ibid.,* 314–315.

32. *Ibid.,* 315–316.

33. *Ibid.,* 311.

34. Interview, R. C. Hogan (WHO), 6 October 1981.

35. WHO/SE/69.1, p. 1.

36. D. A. Henderson, "Smallpox Surveillance in the Strategy of Global Eradication," Inter-regional Seminar on Cholera and Smallpox. Malaysia and Singapore. 11–18 November 1972. WHO/SE/72.8.

37. Interview, J. Donald Millar (CDC), 15 May 1981.

38. Interview, Joel Breman (CDC), 6 May 1981.

39. Interview, Leo Morris (CDC), 13 May 1981.

40. James W. Hicks, "A Review of West African Operations: Methods and Tactics." *The Smallpox Eradication Report,* Vol. 4 (January 1970), 198.

41. Interview, R. C. Hogan (WHO), 6 October 1981.

42. Interview, William Foege (CDC), 13 May 1981.

43. Interview, J. Michael Lane (CDC), 15 May 1981.

44. Interview, Stanley Foster (CDC), 7 May 1981.

45. Interview, Ralph H. Henderson (WHO), 6 October 1981.

46. Interview, R. C. Hogan (WHO), 6 October 1981.

47. David Egli, "Yugoslavia: Conquest of an Epidemic," *World Health* (October 1972), 28–31. See also S. Litvinjenko, B. Arsic, S. Brojanovic, "Epidemiological Aspects of Smallpox in Yugoslavia in 1972." WHO/SE/73.57. See also Bogoljub Arsic and Stevan Litvinjenko, "Smallpox Epidemic in Yugoslavia" (1972), 14 *Yugoslav Survey* (November 1973), 67–74.

48. Interviews, Joel Breman (CDC), 6 May 1981, and J. Michael Lane (CDC), 6 May 1981.

49. Foege himself agrees with this. Interview, William H. Foege (CDC), 13 May 1981.

50. Interview, Jock Copland (WHO), 4 November 1981.

51. Interview, Donald R. Hopkins (CDC), 6 May 1981.

52. Confidential interviews No. 1 and 2.

53. Interview, R. C. Hogan (WHO), 2 December 1981.

54. Letter, D. A. Henderson (WHO) to S. Foster (CDC), 18 August 1976.

55. Interview, William H. Foege (CDC), 14 May 1981.

56. Interview, D. A. Henderson (with Carolyn Buie), March 1979.

57. Interview, Tom Leonard (CDC), 12 May 1981.

58. Interviews, William H. Foege (CDC), 13 May 1981 and J. Michael Lane (CDC), 15 May 1981.

59. Brilliant, *The Management of Smallpox Eradication in India,* pp. 26–27.

60. P. A. Koswara, "Is Routine Vaccination a Necessity in a Smallpox Eradication Programme?" WHO/SE/71.30, p. 121.

61. D. A. Henderson, "Summary—Surveillance," Seminar on Smallpox Eradication and Measles Control in West and Central Africa. Lagos, Nigeria, 13-20 May 1969-Part II.

62. William H. Foege, *et al.,* "Selected Epidemiologic Control . . . ," 315.

63. Interview, I. D. Ladnyi (WHO), 20 November 1981.

64. Interview, A. I. Gromyko (WHO), 20 November 1981.

65. D. A. Henderson, "Surveillance of Smallpox," WHO/SE/75.76, p. 1.

66. See, for example, Stanley O. Foster, *et al.,* "Smallpox Surveillance in Bangladesh: I–Development of Surveillance Containment Strategy," 9 *International Journal of Epidemiology* (1980), 329–334.

67. Surveillance was discussed in WHO Doc. SE/66.3, which set forth the basic approach. The WHO *Handbook for Smallpox Eradication Programmes in Endemic Areas* (SE/67.5, July 1967) explained the concept of "fire-fighting" teams and contained a chapter on surveillance in substantial detail. In Section XI, the concept of target or high-risk groups was discussed.

68. As cited in Brilliant. *The Management of Smallpox Eradication in India,* p. 15.

69. A. D. Langmuir, "The Surveillance of Communicable Diseases of National Importance," 268 *New England Journal of Medicine,* 182–192, quoted by D. A. Henderson, "Surveillance of Smallpox," WHO/SE/75.76, p. 2.

70. D. A. Henderson, "Smallpox in the World." Seminar on Smallpox Eradication, Dacca, 29 October–5 November 1969. WHO/EM/SEM.SE/6, p. 7.

71. Interview, I. D. Ladnyi (WHO), 20 November 1981.

72. D. A. Henderson, "Surveillance of Smallpox," WHO/ES/75.76, pp. 1–2.

73. D. A. Henderson, "The Global Smallpox Eradication Programme—the Final Phase," WHO SE/73.10, p. 3.74. D. A. Henderson, "Summary—Status of the Global Programme." Inter-Regional Seminar on Surveillance and Assessment in Smallpox Eradication. New Delhi, 30 November–5 December 1970. WHO SE/WP/70.1, p. 3.

75. *WHO Expert Committee on Smallpox Eradication: Second Report* (Geneva: WHO, 1972), pp. 9–10.

76. D. A. Henderson, "Epidemiology in the Global Eradication of Smallpox," 1 *International Journal of Epidemiology* (1972), 25.

77. D. A. Henderson, "Surveillance of Smallpox," WHO/SE/75.76, p. 10.

78. WHO, *The Global Eradication of Smallpox* (WHO: Geneva, 1980), p. 31.

79. Brilliant. *The Management of Smallpox Eradication in India,* pp. 11–12.

80. D. A. Henderson, "Smallpox Shows the Way," *World Health* (March 1977), 26.

81. Interview, A. J. R. Taylor (WHO), 2 December 1981.

82. Interview, William H. Foege (CDC), 13 May 1981.

83. *Ibid.*

84. Interview, Joel Breman (CDC), 6 May 1981.

85. Stanley I. Music, "Smallpox Eradication in Bangladesh: Reflections of an Epidemiologist." Unpublished dissertation, London School of Hygiene and Tropical Medicine (1976), p. 26.

86. S. O. Foster, "Smallpox eradication: lessons learned in Bangladesh," 31 *WHO Chronicle* (1977), 245– 247.

87. *Ibid.*

88. S. O. Foster, *et al.,* "Surveillance of Smallpox in Bangladesh . . . ," 329–334.

89. The following discussion relies on P. J. Shrestha, D. A. Robinson, and J. Friedman. *The Nepal Smallpox Eradication Programme* (Kathmandu: H. M. Government of Nepal and WHO, 1977), especially pp. 17–20.

90. H. M. Government of Nepal and WHO. *The Nepal Smallpox Eradication Programme: Description and Analysis* (Kathmandu, 1977), p. 12.

91. P. N. Shrestha, D. A. Robinson, and J. Friedman. *The Nepal Smallpox Eradication Programme: Description and Analysis.* WHO Doc. SME/77.1, 1977, p. 99.

92. *Ibid.,* p. 101.

93. Nepal Smallpox Eradication Project. *Operational Guide for Smallpox Eradication in Nepal from Shrawan 2032 (July 1975).* WHO Doc. SME/77.1, pp. 125-126.

94. *Ibid.,* p. 126.

95. *Expansion of the Use of Immunizations in Developing Countries.* First WHO Seminar, Kumasi, Ghana, 12-19 November 1974. (Geneva: World Health Organization, 1975), pp. 21-30.

96. Arun M. Chacko, "A Goddess Defied," *World Health* (May 1980), 15.

97. Bernard Challenor, "Cultural Resistance to Smallpox Vaccination in West Africa." WHO/SE/68.4.

98. Interview, Tom Leonard (CDC), 12 May 1981.

99. Interview, Z. Jezek (WHO), 15 December 1981.

100. Music, "Smallpox Eradication in Bangdalesh," pp. 35- 38.

101. E. A. Morinis, "Two Pathways in Understanding Disease: Traditional and Scientific," 32 *WHO Chronicle* (1978), 58.

102. *Ibid.,* p. 59.

103. C. G. Pandit, "Local and Social Aspects of the Smallpox Eradication Campaign." WHO/SEA/SPX/Conf. 4.

104. Brilliant. *The Management of Smallpox Eradication in India,* p. 159.

105. S. H. Hassan, "Farewell to Sitala Mayya." WHO Doc. WHO/SE/75.77, p. 5.

106. Interview, Walter Orenstein (CDC), 8 May 1981.

107. P. H. Crippen, "Public Health Administration in a Developing Country: Major Problems Observed in Bangladesh." Unpublished manuscript, 1978(?).

108. Interview, Mary Guinan (CDC), 15 May 1981.

109. Interview, Leo Morris (CDC), 13 May 1981.

110. Interview, Walter Orenstein (CDC), 8 May 1981.

111. *Ibid.*

112. Interview, Stanley Music (CDC), 15 May 1981.

113. Peter Crippin, "Public Health Administration in a Developing Country," p. 6.

114. Interview, Walter Orenstein (CDC), 8 May 1981.

115. Shurkin, *The Invisible Fire,* p. 320.

116. Interview, Jock Copland (WHO), 4 November 1981.

117. Interview, Mary Guinan (CDC), 15 May 1981.

118. S. O. Foster, *et al.,* "Smallpox Surveillance in Bangladesh . . . ," 330-331.

119. Music, "Smallpox Eradication in Bangladesh," pp. 24-25, 31.

120. Interview, Joel Breman (CDC), 8 May 1981.

121. Shurkin, *The Invisible Fire,* p. 339.

122. William J. Siffin, *Problem Analysis: Lessons from a Case of Smallpox,* (Bloomington: Program of Advanced Studies in Institution Building and Technical Assistance Methodology, 1977).

5

Technological Innovation

It is owing to your discovery . . . that in the future the peoples of the world will learn about this disgusting smallpox disease only from ancient traditions.
—Thomas Jefferson to Edward Jenner (1806)

The machine itself makes no demands and holds out no promises: it is the human spirit that makes demands and keeps promises.
—Lewis Mumford

The smallpox eradication campaign may be examined also from a technological perspective; this dimension of the smallpox eradication campaign may be surveyed rather briefly. Technologically, several key advances facilitated the eradication campaign. A strategy of mass vaccination, however feasible it might have been over the long run, depended largely upon efficient delivery techniques and effective vaccines.

The 1959 campaign suffered from inconsistent vaccine quality, among other things. The widely-used liquid vaccine retained its potency for no more than 48 hours and was often contaminated. A major element in the success of the 1966 campaign was efficient, reliable, mass production of potent, stable, *freeze-dried vaccine*. The development of freeze-dried vaccine provides an instructive lesson in appropriate technology. The main work was carried out at the Lister Institute in London and it was accomplished with very limited resources in terms of staff or equipment. The first apparatus for heat-sealing the ampoules of dried vaccine on a production scale was made from a child's toy construction kit. It worked. The Lister Institute made the method freely available and provided exchanges of visiting workers and technicians.[1] Part of the success was due to WHO's agreement with two laboratories (the Rijksinstitut voor de Volkgezondheid in the Netherlands and Connaught Laboratories, Ltd. in Canada) to serve as vaccine reference centers and to provide testing to insure high quality vaccines.[2] As early as 1952, WHO initiated a research program designed to determine the stability of existing dried vaccines and to find a method of production that would produce a consistently stable product. This production method was made available to all countries which requested it, and WHO assisted several countries which planned to begin production of the vaccine.[3] But when WHO began testing in 1967, the quality of donated vaccine was found to be "surprisingly poor and large quantities had to be rejected."

Only one-third of the batches tested at that time met WHO requirements and probably less than 15 percent of the vaccine then used in endemic countries was freeze-dried vaccine meeting WHO requirements.[4]

The testing performed by these labs led to a rapid improvement in the quality of vaccines. Gradually, after sufficient quality controls were regularized, and with technical assistance and equipment provided by WHO, several countries achieved self-sufficiency in vaccine production.

In 1967, WHO conducted a survey of vaccine production capabilities because only limited information was available. By 1969, 58 countries were participating in the production of freeze-dried vaccine; 81 laboratories were either producing or preparing to produce vaccine; 64 were in routine production.

Urgent steps were taken to improve the quality of vaccine. A seminar on vaccine production was conducted in March 1968. Consultation, fellowship training, and independent testing of batches of vaccine were provided. In 1969, the Connaught and Rijksinstitut laboratories were designated as WHO regional reference centers for smallpox vaccine.[5]

Early in the program, a major effort went toward developing more efficient and simpler methodologies for vaccine production, including the preparation of a detailed production manual, better scarification instruments, blueprints for equipment, and other improvements.[6] However, proof of the efficacy of freeze-dried vaccine did not lead immediately to its complete adoption and acceptance. India continued to use liquid vaccine long after freeze-dried vaccine had been adopted in most countries.[7] The low take rates in many instances in India were very probably due to low-potency liquid vaccine. As late as 1967, India still had fourteen vaccine production units producing liquid vaccine and had some 35 million doses of this type on hand.[8] But overall, as Table 5.1 shows, dramatic improvements occurred in the quality of vaccines tested.

The second major technological advance, once dependable freeze-dried vaccines were assured, was the use of the *jet injector.* Before the development of the device, the most common technique for vaccination was the scratch method. A drop of vaccine was scratched into the superficial skin layers, sometimes resulting in serious wounds to the patient, especially when a rotary lancet was employed. Another common method employed a needle which was pressed repeatedly into the skin. Both techniques were deficient for various reasons and were inadequate for mass vaccinations

TABLE 5.1 Vaccine Batches Tested by WHO Reference Centres
Percent with Satisfactory Results

Year	No. of Batches Tested	Percent Satisfactory
1967	73	31
1968	169	58
1969	235	76
1970	412	82
1971	233	77
1972	324	82
1973	400	95
1974	227	92
1975	185	86
1976	245	96
1977	150	93
1978	54	89

Source: WHO. The Global Eradication of Smallpox (Geneva: WHO, 1980), p. 29.

over short time periods. The jet injector (modified for the more superficial smallpox vaccination) provided a means of rapidly vaccinating large numbers of people (over 1,000 vaccinations per hour were possible). The National Communicable Disease Center and the Army Research and Development Command, beginning in 1963, carried out field tests of a hydraulic-powered, foot-actuated, portable jet injector. In inoculations of over 100,000 persons in the United States, Jamaica, Brazil, Tonga, Panama, and Togo, the jet injector's performance exceeded all expectations.

Although the jet injectors were effective under controlled conditions, they presented problems of cost and maintenance. The project staff for the West African campaign searched constantly for means to improve and economize. Alternate sources for spare parts and cleaning kits saved substantial amounts. Special hydraulic fluid for jet injector pumps was replaced by ordinary transmission fluid at a large savings.[9] In areas where house-to-house vaccination was traditional, the jet injector was an expensive device with little compensating advantage. But the jet injector did give impetus to WHO's global smallpox eradication program.

The *bifurcated needle* represented the third major technological advance and it filled a vitally important need in the campaign. Some fifteen years of development went into the bifurcated needle, which was a direct outgrowth of Dryfax, the vaccine developed by Wyeth Laboratories in the late 1950's. The development of freeze-dried vaccine required some new method of vaccine application and use. The classical technique of storage in capillaries was no longer feasible, since the vaccine had to be reconstituted and given in small volumes. This led Wyeth to seek methods to provide single-dose presentations of the stabilized form of the vaccine.

Developed at the Wyeth Laboratories, the two-pronged needle permitted rapid, efficient, and economical vaccinations. Starting in 1961, Benjamin A. Rubin collaborated with Gus Chakros of the Reading Textile Machine Company (now a division of Rockwell International) in needle design. It occurred to Rubin "that a prolonged needle would retain the capillary activity of a loop, and that it might have simultaneous utility in scarification." He suggested the use of a sewing needle in which the loop end was ground down to give a prolonged fork. A piece of wire was cut to the right length, stamped to give the fork shape with dimension to hold exactly one milligram of water by capillarity. A mass tumbling system was used to sharpen the forks of large numbers of needles. ". . . When the bifurcated tip of the needle is dipped into the vaccine, a constant amount is suspended between the prongs, ready for inoculation."[10] A drop of vaccine (suspended between the tines of the needle) is sufficient for a vaccination. Experience showed that one-tenth of the standard vaccine dose in the needle prongs gave equally effective results. *Any* visible amount of vaccine would give the maximum expected response. "This system was therefore found to be quite foolproof."

Extensive tests by Dr. Malcolm Bierly (the first on humans was on juveniles in a detention center in Camp Hill, Pennsylvania) produced "take" rates of 100 percent. Even with vaccine substantially diluted, the needle achieved "takes."[11] Wyeth was granted a patent on the bifurcated needle on 13 July 1965 after prosecution of a case in the Patent Office. Dr. Howard Tint then invented a clever dispenser to allow removal of individual needles from a sterile container without contaminating the other needles.[12] It was found that almost any form of scarification would lead to successful "takes"—even accidental grazing of the skin.[13] Special construction of the needle made it possible to boil or flame it over 200 time without dulling it.[14] The cost of the bifurcated needle was almost nil. One-thousand needles cost only $5.00, and over 100 vaccinations could be done with each needle.[15]

After a relatively short field trial period, the bifurcated needle received enthusiastic approval from the campaign staff:

> In my humble opinion, I would have to rate this as a truly imaginative invention—but, as they say, the simplest devices are often the best and the most frequently overlooked. The bifurcated needle could prove to be

a real boon to the entire programme, its significance ranking in importance with the development of the jet injector.[16]

Extensive studies and tests of the needle were carried out in various locations by field personnel. There were some problems reported (one regional office stated that in 40 percent of the cases, the bifurcated needle was not picking up vaccine from the vial satisfactorily),[17] but generally results were highly successful. It is ironic that some countries, notably India, were slow to adopt the bifurcated needle, in spite of its obvious superiority to devices such as the rotary lancet, which was painful and often left disfiguring scars from the vaccination.[18]

After the extensive field tests, WHO bought hundreds of thousands of the bifurcated needles and used them in the field, starting in Zaire in 1968. WHO also got free rights to manufacture the needle. A decision by Wyeth that other parties who bought the needle would have to buy Dryfax with it led to a long dispute between Wyeth and WHO regarding sales of the needle. Many countries had developed independent capability for producing vaccine and had no intention of buying it from Wyeth, even if this meant forgoing the bifurcated needle. After protracted exchange of correspondence between Henderson and Wyeth officials, in May 1972 Wyeth agreed to sell the needles without the vaccine, and ended up making very little profit, because of WHO manufacturing rights.[19]

Experience gained as the campaign progressed demonstrated another more efficient approach to vaccination. Standard practice had been to swab the patient's vaccination site with acetone, soap, or alcohol before vaccination. Studies showed that such cleansing made no significant difference in terms of bacterial infection. As a result, the field teams were able to simplify the vaccination technique further by reducing the time required and the amount of supplies to be carried.

Without detracting at all from the vital contribution of each of these technological factors, I would observe only that except for dramatic improvements in vaccine quality control, none of the developments was directly the result of the smallpox eradication campaign itself. It is true that the campaign afforded an opportunity to test the bifurcated needle under a variety of conditions and that these tests led to improvement of the needle. The most critical technological contribution of the campaign, however, appears to have been its promotion of the capacity to produce high quality vaccine in many countries. Indeed, a major part of the initial work of the Smallpox Eradication Unit in WHO was given over to vaccine production and quality control; this task was assigned the highest priority as a *sina qua non* of the campaign.

The successful application of technology in the smallpox eradication campaign reminds us again of the critical role of management in the overall process. Jenner's vaccination technique was almost universally understood as a reliable preventive of smallpox. Adequate tools for vaccination were available and the technology for production of effective vaccine were in place well before the worldwide eradication campaign began. Yet the essential linchpins, which were determined management and the dedication to see it through, were lacking until 1966. Then the best of technology, management skills, and human spirit combined to change the world dramatically.

Notes

1. L. H. Collier, "Appropriate Technology in the Development of Freeze-dried Smallpox Vaccine," 34 *WHO Chronicle* (1980), 179.
2. Donald A. Henderson, "The Eradication of Smallpox," 235 *Scientific American* (October 1976), 29.
3. WHO Doc. EB21/WP/21, 24 January 1958, pp. 3–4.
4. I. Arita, "The Control of Vaccine Quality in the Smallpox Eradication Programme," 19 *Standard* (1972), 79.
5. I. Arita and D. A. Henderson, "Freeze-dried Vaccine for the Smallpox Eradication Program." Seminar on Smallpox Eradication, Dacca, 29 October–5 November 1969. WHO/EM/SEM.SE/38, pp. 3–4.
6. Donald A. Henderson, "Smallpox Shows the Way," *World Health* (March 1977), 24.
7. Lawrence B. Brilliant, *The Management of Smallpox Eradication in India* (Ann Arbor: The University of Michigan Press, 1985), p. 79.
8. *Ibid.*, p. 15.
9. James W. Hicks, "A Review of West African Operations; Methods and Tactics." *The SEP Report,* Vol 4. (January 1970), 194.
10. B. A. Rubin, "A Note on the Development of the Bifurcated Needle for Smallpox Vaccination," 34 *WHO Chronicle* (1980), 180–181.
11. Joel N. Shurkin, *The Invisible Fire,* Ch. XII.
12. Letter, B. A. Rubin (Wyeth Laboratories) to J. S. Copeland (WHO), 12 December 1974.
13. Letter, B. A. Rubin (Wyeth Laboratories) to I. Arita (WHO), 31 December 1979.
14. Henderson, "The Eradication of Smallpox," 30.
15. WHO/SE/71.30, p. 227.
16. Letter, D. A. Henderson (WHO) to Dr. Malcolm Bierley (Wyeth Laboratories), 8 March 1967.
17. Letter, S. Falkland to I. D. Ladnyi, 9 July 1968. See also I. D. Ladnyi, "Studies of Smallpox Vaccination by Bifurcated Needles in Kenya." WHO SE/68.7.
18. Brilliant, *The Management of Smallpox Eradication in India,* p. 79.
19. Shurkin, *The Invisible Fire,* Ch. XII.

6

Program Evaluation and Assessment

The World Health Organization, well in advance of the second eradication campaign, had foreseen the critical role of evaluation:

> In all campaigns concurrent evaluation is as essential as the final assessment
> of the programme. The evaluation should be carried out by independent
> teams to discover defects in time to remedy them while the programme
> is still active.[1]

As in many other aspects of the eradication program, procedures for
program evaluation and assessment constantly evolved as experience
accrued. This gradual refinement of the evaluation system required not
only a recasting of the highest level goal but also the development of
ever more precise and realistic measures of performance.

James E. Austin has stressed the importance of certain characteristics
of goal setting that are essential if they are to be useful in on-going
and later program evaluation. He emphasizes that goals should be specific,
measurable, realistic, and dynamic.[2] The original goals of the smallpox
eradication program, as envisioned by the WHO expert committees and
by the World Health Assembly, were quite specific, but not realistic.
Their realism was suspect both because of unreliable data on smallpox
incidence and their feasibility. It fell to the Smallpox Eradication Unit,
using the dramatic successes of the Nigerian campaign, to redefine the
goals in realistic terms that lent themselves to useful program evaluation.
Program managers were adamant about keeping the evaluation and
assessment measures flexible and dynamic, so that they could be tailored
to each particular environment. Initial measures, such as the number of
people vaccinated, proved to be not useful, and were replaced by trends
in the incidence of smallpox. Though this was useful as a macro-level
measure, greater specificity was required at lower levels. Thus in India
in 1974, attention turned to outbreaks pending in infected areas; in
1975, the outcome of surveillance searches was the focus, and finally,

as the campaign appeared successful, search efficiency was emphasized. Tactics to implement the goals also underwent a gradual process of increasing specificity. The 1970 plan of operations in India called for mass vaccination whenever an outbreak was discovered. By 1973, this had changed to focus on finding as many hidden cases as possible and then vaccinating 30 households closest to each infected house. In early 1974, the radius was extended to cover 50 households, and later, vaccination of the entire village and posting of two watchguards were employed. Eventually, the search area was broadened to 16 kilometers around the infected house and saturation vaccination of everyone within 1.6 kilometers was carried out.[3]

One of the most difficult and least efficient links in the surveillance program was the development of procedures for routine reporting of smallpox cases. Many cases were not reported because of simple lack of interest or the expectation or knowledge that no action or assistance would result. Other cases were cared for at home and never brought to the attention of medical personnel. In some countries, notably India, reporting of cases even brought reprimands from higher officials. Accurate data collection and dissemination formed the most critical element of the overall control system. Henderson observed that ". . . surprising problems were initially encountered . . ." in the efforts to establish procedures. The difficulty was not unique to a particular country or region, although a disproportionate number of references to the problem relate to India:

> When the joint WHO-government of India Plan of Operations of 1970 recommitted India to the goal of eradication, the reported incidence of smallpox was decreasing. But the measurement tool—the reporting system—was not accurate. The apparent effectiveness of the program was an illusion that was shattered when increasingly accurate measurement uncovered a high number of unreported cases, raising reported smallpox cases to seemingly epidemic levels. Before 1970, the NSEP [National Smallpox Eradication Program] was neither making effective progress toward the final goal of eradication or even adequately defining the problem so that measurable targets could be set."[4]

In a 1966 report, WHO had cautioned against the use of simple measurement of the number of vaccinations given:

> Measurement of the proportion of a population vaccinated may be useful as a guide with respect to the conduct of a programme. However, it must be kept in mind that such measurement represents a guide only and the actual success of the programme must be appraised in terms of the disappearance of the disease. Although a certain high proportion of the

population may have been vaccinated in principle, it must be recognized that substantially less are actually successfully vaccinated. Further, an overall indication of coverage rate says nothing regarding the distribution of vaccination.

. . . The ultimate measure of any eradication programme is its success in reducing the number of cases to zero. So long as the disease is endemically transmitted, an eradication programme has failed to achieve its goal whatever the proportion of the population apparently successfully vaccinated.[5]

A serious problem was the need to break away from a system in which an isolated statistical unit processed all health data, without real responsibility or working contact with the rest of the health ministry or health care system. Such units tended to hold reports until all reports from an area had been received and did not consider it their responsibility to assure that all reports were received. Almost never did such units question unusual reports. Henderson found that reports at higher levels often were misleading and the number of cases tended to diminish at each level. In one instance, 100 cases at the sub-district level evaporated to 70 in the district report, 40 at the provincial level, and finally to 25 registered in the national report. On occasion, deliberate suppression of reports occurred, but more often the cause was inept data processing. For this reason, the Smallpox Eradication Unit gave high priority to the establishment of reporting control and program evaluation and insisted that program officers assume primary responsibility for smallpox case reporting.[6] Experience showed that reporting improved rapidly when special assistance was provided promptly. Many forms of "feedback" were employed at different levels of the program as a means of exchanging information and keeping staff informed. Various types of newsletters and similar devices were used in most countries for this purpose, and then proved to be invaluable. For example, a monthly newsletter, "The Eradicator," was published by project staff in Sierra Leone.

Program evaluation indicators were changed with experience and methods were refined gradually as the organization learned. In Asia, in general, evaluation was based ultimately on the ability to document the absence of smallpox by completeness of searches and specimens taken.[7]

However, different critical indicators were employed at various periods during the ten-year campaign to evaluate program success. The indicators changed progressively from a rather crude measure such as the number of vaccinations (India, to suggest the problem, had vaccinated a number of persons equal to approximately twice its population), to percentage of coverage, cases and deaths, number of infected villages, the surveillance interval (representing the time between the first case and the date of detection), and containment (the time between detection and the last case. Containment was judged effective when no new cases occurred after 15 days). In each situation, failures were analyzed and corrective action taken. In later assessment efforts, key questions determined respondents' knowledge of the reward and location for case reporting, the assumption being that such knowledge would almost surely result in reports.[8]

In Brazil, it was estimated that only some two percent of the smallpox cases in that country were ever reported. Indeed, there was virtually no national reporting system for any disease when the smallpox program commenced. "Reports were received on an irregular, often annual basis, and usually pertained to cases occurring in the state capitals only." An urgent early task was the establishment of a reporting system. That effort proved to be complicated because of Brazil's federal organization, but by the second year, the system was functioning and it gradually expanded. By the end of 1969, all but two states were reporting weekly to the *Campanha de Erradicação da Variola* (CEV).[9]

Once in place, the reporting system provided a basis for independent judgment concerning the incidence of smallpox. As expected, a functional reporting system increased the number of cases reported and, as later in India, caused problems in terms of convincing public health and political officials that the eradication campaign was achieving its objectives.[10]

Program evaluation in Brazil was expanded steadily to the point where assessment surveys were carried out seven days after smallpox eradication teams passed through an area. This form of assessment provided an independent check on take rates and encouraged honest performance by teams.

Initially, the Brazilian program director was reluctant to allocate funds to evaluation. But in June and July 1967, an outbreak of 51 cases occurred in Branquinhas, Alagoas, after the campaign swept through the area. A special investigating team sent to the region concluded that either poor reporting or lies about the extent of vaccination had occurred. When a random sample of the population revealed that only 55 percent had been vaccinated—instead of the 100 percent reported—the eradication team and its supervisor were fired. The situation in Alagoas persuaded the director to provide funds for concurrent evaluation and the work of the assessment teams was publicized widely.[11] (The Alagoas episode demonstrated the problems that could occur in the campaign without independent concurrent assessment.)

Program evaluation, as the worldwide campaign matured organizationally, became more systematic and comprehensive. Reports became gradually more specific and detailed; target times were set and used; and indicators were clear and revealing. Surveys after vaccination teams passed through an area were based on systematic random sampling, and of course, the "proof of the pudding" was smallpox incidence.[12]

In Sierra Leone, from 1968, coverage and take rates were assessed routinely by probability samplings of about five percent of the inhabitants of each chiefdom, some six to eight days after vaccination. Samples were biased deliberately to include a higher proportion of persons from villages beyond vaccination centers.[13]

Millar, as a result of the West Africa campaign, defined the fundamental objectives of assessment as follows:

1. to determine if the population is being reached
2. to determine whether those being reached are being immunized (referring to "take rates")
3. to determine why this is so
4. to initiate corrective action based on the assessment

Assessment in West Africa revealed, among other things, that overall coverage was lower than expected in most countries. The frequency of smallpox scars increased with age, as expected. But the most dramatic point was how rapidly the immune population under the age of one was "diluted." Unvaccinated susceptibles among the newborn rapidly lowered the level of immunity. Clearly, greater efforts to reach this group were required if the reservoir necessary to support smallpox transmission was to be eliminated.[14]

In Afghanistan, after the mass vaccination program began in 1969, a systematic concurrent assessment procedure was evolved and used, because "it was suspected that the vaccination figures were, in many instances, fictitious." A team of five assessors headed by a sanitarian assessed the work of five or six vaccination teams. They were chosen specially from among the best vaccinators. Assessment basically focused on surveying scars from vaccination, variolation, or smallpox itself, and the survey was performed on a continuing basis in a sample of areas. The zonal director chose 30–40 percent of the localities, either by drawing lots or using a table of random numbers. Each individual was checked first for pockmarks, then a variolation scar, then a vaccination scar, or a recent vaccination take, in that order. The work of the assessment teams was checked also (one team in the Kabul area was dismissed for filling out forms without actually conducting the survey.)[15]

After a recurrence of smallpox in Nigeria (1970), William Foege drew several implications from the investigations:

• A mass vaccination program is not sufficient in itself to eradicate smallpox.

- The absence of reports should not be interpreted to mean the absence of disease.
- If assessments are to be worthwhile they must result in corrective action.
- Increased emphasis on surveillance should take place when an area is believed to be free from smallpox. "Transmission at low levels and in remote areas has been repeatedly observed. A high index of suspicion is required to find these foci before they become larger epidemics."
- "The value of an investigation cannot be over-estimated. A single case of smallpox in this instance led to the discovery of four outbreaks with a total of 75 cases of smallpox."[16]

The Nigerian smallpox/measles program plan of operations for Fiscal Year 1971 (by which time the campaign was stabilizing its plan of attack) provided for four types of assessment for program evaluation:

1. *Supervisory assessment* checked individual performance by assessing a village vaccinated by a team one week previously. Coverage and take rates were measured.
2. *Area assessment,* using a cluster sample technique, focused on the immunity level of completed areas.
3. *Maintenance assessment* determined coverage of the target age groups (primarily 6–18 months and 18–36 months).
4. *Special assessments* determined immunity in the area of smallpox endemicity and evaluated effectiveness of control procedure.[17]

In India, the National Commission for Assessment of the Smallpox Eradication Programme, set up to assess the campaign results in that country, examined the following factors during its visits:

- the awareness of the population concerning the necessity to report smallpox cases promptly, if they occurred, and to where they should be reported
- evidence of publicity and knowledge of the 1,000 rupees reward for reporting cases
- pockmark survey to discover any evidence of cases not previously notified
- the investigation of any current outbreak involving fever with fresh cases or reports of a case difficult to diagnose
- the quality of epidemiological investigation done by local staff[18]

After July 1975 in Nepal, routine assessment of active surveillance activities was carried out by use of a questionnaire administered by district supervisors in their own districts and by the two national assessment teams. The assessment was designed to give reliable information on two factors: (1) whether surveillance teams had been working in the district, and (2) whether the public awareness of the reward and appropriate action to be taken was at such a level that cases of smallpox would be brought to the attention of the authorities if they occurred.

For these purposes, four questions were asked:

1. Have you seen anybody recently inquiring about smallpox cases?
2. Has anybody shown you the smallpox recognition card recently?
3. Do you know about the reward offered for information about smallpox?
4. Do you know where to report any case of smallpox you hear about?[19]

In Bangladesh, the control system emphasized *failure analysis*. At a monthly meeting at either the regional or national level, team leaders examined breakdowns in the surveillance system and attempted to understand them.[20]

When the final campaign geared up in 1975, the goal was to find at least 80 percent of the cases within 15 days after an attack—100 percent containment was expected within 21 days of detection. At least 90 percent of all cases were to be traced to the source. A health worker was assigned to each infected village and guards were posted at infected houses. Tally forms were used to insure that everyone in a half-mile radius was vaccinated.[21] In the infected village surveillance strategy, the goal was to detect every infected village within 14 days of occurrence of the first case in the village.[22]

Surveillance and Special Assessment: India

In India, as the campaign was approaching success, special assessment surveys were used in remote areas to detect "weak spots" in local smallpox eradication programs that required remedial action. The objectives were (1) to assess effectiveness of local eradication activities; (2) to assess epidemiological data showing the history of smallpox transmission in selected localities; and (3) to assess the vaccination status of selected samples of the population.

Data were collected by a team consisting of an experienced medical officer and a health supervisor. Questions included demographic data

(age, sex, ethnic group, and language) in addition to detailed information on recent or previous vaccinations.
Several specific questions were asked about the history of smallpox:

1. Has there ever been a case of smallpox in your household? In what year did this occur?
2. Have you ever seen a case of smallpox in your neighboring block? Where? In which year?
3. If you have never seen a case of smallpox, have you ever heard of someone in your district getting smallpox in your neighboring block? Where? In what year?

Each respondent was asked if he knew of recent search activities, if he had ever seen the smallpox recognition card, if he knew about the 1,000 rupees reward, and if he knew where to report suspected smallpox cases (those with fever and rash).[23]

Searches at weekly markets in India proved to be an effective form of surveillance, but not as effective as the house-to-house method. Reasonably good results were obtained when the search was planned in advance and closely supervised by a medical officer and special search team. Market search required only one-fourth to one-third of the manpower required for house-to-house search. Market search was useful for rapid but not precise evaluation of disease incidence or presence of the disease in the past.[24]

Near the end of the Indian campaign, from June to December 1974, the most critical assessment index was the infected village. This active focus was called a "pending outbreak," meaning that any case in the village "had an onset date recent enough to be considered still potentially infective itself or the source of infection for an incubating case." If at the end of a four (later six) week period no new cases had been found in the village, it was removed from the list of pending outbreaks.[25] Brilliant also discusses the use of "surrogates for smallpox" as an assessment index. Since some villages would report chickenpox as smallpox in the hope of earning the 1,000 rupee reward, in the absence of chickenpox reports in a district, smallpox evaluators would attempt to discover why. The absence of chickenpox reports sometimes indicated poor coverage by search workers, the publicity campaign, or containment teams.[26]

The "infected village" or "pending outbreaks" index became more important toward the end of the Indian campaign, because this provided a means of measuring the active foci that were potentially capable of transmitting the smallpox virus. If several villages widely separated were found to be infected, rather than simply more cases in one village, the implications for resource allocation were very significant.[27] Changes were instituted also in the assessment of vaccine delivery in India. As vaccine quality improved steadily (by 1975, most vaccine produced in India tested potent in WHO reference centers), the number of people vaccinated became less important. Instead, surveys of take-rates in the field provided the best test of vaccine delivery as well as vaccine potency.[28]

Refinement of Surveillance and Containment Strategy

At every stage of the eradication campaign, the basic strategy of surveillance and containment was constantly refined in order to achieve control of the disease through careful quality control. Brilliant observes that in India there was continual assessment after the middle of 1974, to discover deficiencies in containment, determine optimal rates of vaccination so as to minimize secondary spread, and optimal radii of immunity. When known outbreaks disappeared, intensified surveillance was emphasized and assessment focus shifted to the efficacy of surveillance. Search strategy was expanded so that search workers did more than inquire about rash-with-fever cases and show a recognition card; they were also to announce rewards, tell people where to report smallpox cases, and give progress reports to villages. The performance of search workers was evaluated carefully by means of interviews of villagers. Where feedback was negative—that is, when assessment showed that a district did not meet minimal targets, the whole search and assessment process was repeated until results were acceptable. The operation called "Smallpox Zero" worked, and on 24 May 1975, the last known smallpox case in India was discovered.[29]

The Indian campaign shows another example of management innovation in program evaluations. Normally, in statistical analysis of a population, a random sample would be employed to derive general information. But the program staff in India, in order to determine the public's awareness of the rewards for reporting of smallpox cases, used skewed samples instead of random samples. This enabled the survey to be focused on areas where other forms of assessment suggested that problems existed. People who did not know about the reward were more important to the eradication effort than those who did know. "Preferential assessment of the weakest link was a good supervision strategy in this case."[30]

Operation Smallpox Zero: India

As the number of cases diminished in India, health workers tended to become complacent, a problem that Henderson saw as the "greatest danger." Operation Smallpox Zero was intended to consolidate the victory and to maintain surveillance up to May 1977. The main techniques employed were periodic active search operations; surveillance at markets, fairs, festivals, hospitals, and outdoor clinics; and special surveillance in selected areas of high risk.

High risk areas were defined as:

- remote areas that may be missed by regular searches
- areas recently affected by smallpox infection
- border areas which attract visitors from neighboring countries
- areas which are cut off by seasonal changes
- areas of pilgrimage, fairs, and festivals
- areas where health staff are absent or no one has taken the responsibility
- areas with beggars and nomads
- areas having seasonal workers, transient population, and low socio-economic groups
- other vulnerable areas such as coal mines, char areas, refugee camps, and construction sites

Other techniques used in Operation Smallpox Zero were continuous surveillance by surveillance teams, continuous routine surveillance by all health staff, fever and rash case outbreak surveillance, a secondary surveillance system, publicity about the smallpox reward, and routine notification and regular reporting.[31]

Nicole Grasset points to the most wearying task in India as

> fighting against delays. We were constantly battling against time, as areas free of smallpox in Asia were constantly in danger of being re-infected by the highly endemic regions; so we had to act rapidly. We always set a specific time limit to any operation.[32]

Brilliant likens the two-year intensive vigil from 1975 to 1977, necessary for certifying eradication in India, as the "realm of the final inch," or the last, excruciating struggle to attain perfection in the eradication task.[33] He quotes another participant as observing that eradication "demanded perfection in detail and compulsive attention to specific tasks."[34]

Notes

1. "Organization of a Smallpox Eradication Campaign," WHO/Smallpox/20, 25 May 1964, p. 3.

2. James E. Austin, *The Management Bottleneck in Family Planning Programs* (Cambridge: Harvard University Graduate School of Business Administration,

1979), cited in Brilliant, *The Management of Smallpox Eradication in India*, p. 83.

3. Brilliant, *The Management of Smallpox Eradication in India*, pp. 84–85.

4. *Ibid.*, p. 125.

5. WHO Doc. A19/P&B/2, 28 March 1966, p. 107–108.

6. D. A. Henderson, "Surveillance of Smallpox," WHO/SE/75.76, pp. 6–7.

7. Interview, Joel Breman (CDC), 8 May 1981.

8. Interview, Stanley O. Foster (CDC), 7 May 1981.

9. Eurico Suzart de Carvalho Filho *et al.*, "Smallpox Eradication in Brazil, 1967–69," 43 *Bulletin of the World Health Organization* (1970), 798.

10. Interview, Leo Morris (CDC), 13 May 1981.

11. *Ibid.* See also Leo Morris, A. Vera Martinez, Jose Oswaldo da Silva, "Epidemiological Investigation of a Smallpox Outbreak in a City Reported to be 100 percent Vaccinated," SE/72.6.

12. Interview, Donald R. Hopkins (CDC), 6 May 1981.

13. WHO/SE/71.30, p. 34.

14. J. D. Millar, "Summary Concurrent Assessment," *The SEP Report* Vol. 4 (January 1970), 133–135.

15. WHO/SE/71.30, pp. 98–101.

16. *Ibid.*, p. 47.

17. Nigerian Smallpox/Measles Program. *Plan of Operations, FY 1971.*

18. R. N. Basu and L. N. Khodakevich, "The National Commission for Assessment of the Smallpox Eradication Programme in India," 22 *Indian Journal of Public Health* (Jan.-Mar. 1978), 19.

19. P. N. Shrestha, D. A. Robinson, and J. Friedman, *The Nepal Smallpox Eradication Programme*, Kathmandu (H.M. Government of Nepal and WHO, 1977), pp. 69–71.

20. Joel Shurkin, *The Invisible Fire*, p. 358.

21. *Ibid.*, p. 362.

22. S. O. Foster, *et al.*, "Smallpox Surveillance in Bangladesh . . . ," 330.

23. Z. Jezek, R. R. Arora, Z. S. Arya, and Zaffar Hussain, "Smallpox Surveillance in Remote and Inaccessible Areas of India," WHO/SE/76.79, p. 1.

24. R. N. Basu and L. N. Khodakevich, "Surveillance at Weekly Markets in the Smallpox Eradication Programme in India," WHO/SE/77.94, p. 4.

25. Brilliant, *The Management of Smallpox Eradication in India*, p. 54.

26. *Ibid.*, pp. 55–56.

27. *Ibid.*, pp. 58–59.

28. *Ibid.*, p. 103.

29. *Ibid.*, pp. 65–68.

30. *Ibid.*, p. 120.

31. Z. Jezek and R. N. Basu, "Operation Smallpox Zero," WHO/SE/76.80, pp. 1–5.

32. N. Grasset, "Faith and Determination," *World Health* (August-September 1976), 38.

33. Brilliant, *The Management of Smallpox Eradication in India,* p. 68. The analogy to A. Solzhenitsyn's "rule of the final inch," in *The First Circle,* was suggested by Professor Holger Lundbeck.

34. *Ibid.,* p. 92.

7

Lessons for the Future

The smallpox eradication campaign "taught the world that frail human beings can plan a rational health future."
—Norman Cousins, 1976

By almost any measure, the eradication of smallpox from the world is a magnificent achievement, one probably unequaled in the history of medicine and public health. Probably no other accomplishment in the ancient struggle against disease exceeds the importance of the final eradication of smallpox.

The eradication campaign recorded the last cases of smallpox in South America and in West and Central Africa in 1971; in Indonesia in 1972; in southern Africa in 1973; and in the Asian subcontinent in 1975. The last known case (of natural origin) occurred in southern Somalia in October 1977.[1]

In a critically important follow-up action to the eradication campaign, WHO decided to undertake an international effort to certify the disease's eradication. Two years after the last known case, an international commission was convened to examine the documentary evidence of eradication and to evaluate it, in part by personal field observations. A major effort by host countries preceded the work of the international commission: routine reporting systems were evaluated; special mobile teams conducted active searches; pockmark surveys were carried out; careful surveillance of chickenpox cases was emphasized; rumor registers were established to monitor and follow-up on all reports of smallpox cases; specimens were collected from patients with chickenpox, persons with fever and rash, and other suspects, and these were sent for laboratory diagnosis; and extensive publicity was given to available rewards (up to $1,000 offered by WHO) for reporting of previously undetected cases. Finally, in December 1979, the Global Commission concluded that smallpox had been eradicated and made several recommendations regarding WHO policy for the future.

We must be cautious about the transferability of any conclusions or lessons drawn from the smallpox eradication campaign, but there are several generalizations of value.

In many respects, the campaign was a triumph of management as much as it was a dramatic technical effort in epidemiology. Indeed the director-general of WHO, Dr. H. Mahler, described the campaign as "a triumph of management, not of medicine." Others, in searching for the keys to understanding the success of the campaign, have focused on a variety of factors. These range from the role of total dedication by people to strong commitment by WHO and governments. They sometimes point to the central role of research and technology—the production of stable, potent, freeze-dried vaccine; the jet injector; and the bifurcated needle. Leadership is identified by others as the prime ingredient, an especially important factor when things went badly. Some believe a certain management approach, including management by objectives, superb reporting and followup, and rigorous evaluation and assessment, was the most important key. It has also been concluded that the key to the campaign's success was the disease itself—smallpox, a highly visible, detectable, controllable disease was appropriate for the application of epidemiologic techniques. Other explanations, such as public involvement, international cooperation, sufficient resources, and a field-oriented staff, have been offered by both participants and observers.

Surely all of these factors, in various ways, contributed to the achievements of the campaign and facilitated the program. A more productive approach to the question, however, might be to concentrate on some of the lessons to be learned from the experience. Following that, it will be useful to speculate about the effects of the smallpox eradication campaign before any general observations and conclusions are reached. That is the purpose of the following section.

Lessons

What, then, might be concluded from the experience? *First,* an organization setting out to attack a problem should strive to insure that the problem has been defined clearly and that objectives and strategies are not confused so that the definition is beclouded. In this case, the problem (or objective) was to eradicate smallpox. Yet that objective, for practical purposes, was recast initially as mass vaccination. This redefinition of the problem in the minds of many—from *eradication of smallpox* to *mass vaccination*—operated so as to delay the organization's focusing on the real problem. This confusion of means and ends, even though the basic campaign strategy after 1968 shifted quite rapidly to surveillance-containment, continued to have profound effects on the campaign. It is probably no exaggeration to say that the confusion of means and ends prevented some governments, organizations, and people from ever fully accepting and supporting the revised strategy. However, once there was unmistakable empirical evidence to support the new strategy, the campaign managers were freer to move resolutely in implementing surveillance-containment throughout the endemic areas of the world. And WHO, to its credit, energetically promoted the new strategy.

Second, understand the enemy, in this case the target, smallpox. The campaign gradually defined the enemy more precisely as experience accumulated. Many long-accepted perceptions of smallpox and its epidemiology were proven incorrect or inadequate—its contagiousness, the rapidity of its spread, its seasonality, etc. An effective organization must be capable of careful observation of events and data and willing to use that knowledge for necessary shifts in strategy and tactics. This is possible only if the target is understood fully in all its characteristics. A corollary lesson should alert planners to the danger of overreliance on traditional expertise. Several of the early conclusions of the WHO expert committees were proven wrong during the campaign.

Third, pick good people. Delegate to high performance staff, using them to the fullest. Selection of staff--people of the highest integrity, knowledge and education, and with the willingness and ability to work under difficult field conditions—should be among the primary concerns of organizational leadership. Nicole Grasset summed it up well:

> The basic element of success in any field is to get good people—the right people. . . . A vacant post is better than having it filled with the wrong person. The qualities they needed, rather than past experience, were faith in their work, courage and perseverance, adaptability to any situation, imagination, efficiency, capacity to take on responsibility yet flexibility to work easily as part of a team, and last but not least, willingness to work hard.[2]

A very important corollary is flexibility in the use of those people. The campaign was successful in part because it employed people according to their abilities, not simply according to normal practice. The use of public health advisers in place of regular M.D.'s is a case in point. As one participant put it, the campaign was a "a victory for sound epidemiology" but also "an enormous amount of slogging" by non-medical workers.[3]

Over and over again, the importance of human qualities was emphasized by participants in the campaign.

> We tend to overemphasize the importance of physical resources. The smallpox programme was based on an unusual combination of human qualities of

an immaterial character, unassailable ethics, strong engagement and excellent intellectual capacity. The chain of ethos-pathos-logos, if you remember. I believe this is the basic reason why so many obstacles such as religious beliefs, political disagreements, administrative inefficiency, indifference, personal craving for power and influence and a number of other human weaknesses could be surmounted.[4]

Throughout the smallpox eradication campaign, there was a strong management commitment to recruit the best staff possible and let them work in their own way. D. A. Henderson was extremely careful, on key posts, to get people in whom he had confidence.[5]

Fourth, build an organization—perhaps better, assemble an organism— that above all retains the capacity to interpret experience and to weigh evidence with the maximum degree of openness, and to respond to that experience and evidence. Much of this capacity stems from a flexible mode of management that encourages and provides a felicitous environment for organizational learning and innovation. A corollary management task must be creative but insistent iconoclasm, to insure that organization members do not begin to reify beliefs and deify conventional modes and objectives. "A key task of administrators . . .is to facilitate the learning capacities of the unit for which they are responsible."[6]

The management of the smallpox campaign proved itself willing and able to recognize that means and ends had been confused in the original problem definition; to experiment with the new strategy of surveillance-containment and to enthusiastically adopt it as the guiding strategy; to adopt a simple technology in the form of the bifurcated needle when a more complex technology—the jet injector—could not do the job; and to constantly search for effective, direct means of assessment.

Fifth, promote an organic capacity in the organization that allows programs, projects, and people to adapt and conform to the imperatives of the task environment. In international efforts such as the smallpox eradication campaign, such adaptation to an infinitely complex mosaic of cultures, religions, health systems, and governmental structures was absolutely essential.

Among other things, this lesson relates to the role of traditional medicine:

the therapeutic strategies utilized by followers of traditional medicine systems are based on genuine beliefs and expectations relating to the body-mind-spirit complex. People will use logic, but not necessarily scientific and empirical logic, in assessing the suitability of various available therapies to satisfy their bodily and other needs. Failure of health planners to consider the role of indigenous medical practice may undermine the operation of any programme, because of its rejection by the people despite its efficacy and scientific validity.[7]

The teams in Bangladesh found that although people generally accepted smallpox as a fact of life to be accepted, when staff effectiveness in controlling it improved, public attitudes changed and cooperation increased along with that.[8] In sum, a quick, flexible response must be available to adapt to local situations and action must be tailored accordingly.

Sixth, provide incentives—both material and organizational incentives—that hold out positive inducements to performance and also facilitate accurate, rather than "good" or "expected" reporting and performance. Avoid organizational arrangements that force members into conflicting roles and that serve to distort interpretation of evidence and faithful performance. A major factor is the use of positive feedback to maintain confidence in the field. The smallpox campaign strived to build close communication among all participants. Frequent visits by headquarters staff encouraged excellent motivation, assisted national program officers, and established high priority for the smallpox campaign.

The campaign's incentives ranged from financial rewards for reporting, to immediate questioning of inaccurate or inconsistent reporting, and modification of organizational structure to separate the surveillance and containment functions in order to minimize the temptation of inaccurate reporting.

Seventh, identify and establish unambiguous, primary, and direct measures of task achievement as the heart of program evaluation. In the smallpox campaign, it would have been easy for managers to focus upon indirect or secondary measures of performance, such as the number of vaccinations given, or the number of teams involved, or the funds expended. The *critical* measure, however, was trends in the incidence of smallpox and that was chosen as the principal index of achievement. *All else was indirect—sometimes even irrelevant.* Managers often fall into the trap of equating effort with results, or inputs with outputs, evaluating programs on the basis of how much goes into them rather than what they achieve.

Henderson speculated, as the campaign entered its fifth year, about the use of appropriate measures of achievement in other programs:

> One wonders if in coping with other preventable infectious diseases, it might not be more productive to expand greater effort on the development of a surveillance programme to monitor what one is actually achieving in reducing morbidity and to redirect as necessary the operation of an otherwise decerebrate mass vaccination programme.[9]

This is not to say that other measures of program performance are not important. Careful assessment of take rates, villages served, number of vaccinations, potential outbreaks, and similar factors must be evaluated. As one participant urged, "evaluate everything—the sooner the better," but he meant evaluation to determine whether an activity contributed to the ultimate objective, eradication of smallpox. There seems to be no alternative to establishment of clear, quantifiable goals and measures for effective management control. Setting quantifiable targets assisted management directly in pinpointing shortfalls and critical gaps and in analyzing failures. Thus the surveillance target in Bangladesh was to detect 80 percent of new outbreaks within 15 days of the first rash in the first outbreak. The containment target was to stop 100 percent of outbreaks in 15 days. It is also important that objectives and measures be expressed simply so that every participant understands what is to be done and his/her role in that effort. The headquarters staff attempted especially to develop an effective communication and feedback system to reinforce individual participation.

Eighth, recognize the importance of details and learn to use them for control and feedback without permitting them to overwhelm the operations. Henderson and Foege were generally acknowledged to be masters in terms of using detailed data and even making data interesting in proving points. The WHO headquarters (not the Smallpox Eradication Unit) was criticized frequently for not coming down to "nitty-gritty" details and coping with them. The smallpox campaign excelled in careful planning and administration. A cardinal rule was: never assume—verify.[10] This attitude permeated the whole organization and paid great dividends. Foege clearly recognized the importance of paperwork and created "systems within systems" in India for control as a result of problems.[11] Yet forms were kept simple and contained only the essential minimum for assessment. This was combined with a regular feedback system to make the data useful. There were periodic review meetings at all levels for exchange of information, analysis of failure, and resolution of problems.

Ninth, seek simplicity. "The smallpox eradication program demonstrated the importance of discipline and simplicity in effective implementation of programs."[12] The bifurcated needle, an utterly simple and inexpensive device, is only one of the examples. It replaced the far more complicated jet injector as the principal tool in field vaccinations. Simple devices, simple procedures, and simple instructions are especially critical in programs where large numbers of people are involved in tasks that demand disciplined performance—as good epidemiology does. Uncomplicated technology and straight-forward procedures lend themselves far more effectively to success in high pressure situations under difficult conditions. An added advantage is the far lower cost in resources. The search for simplicity often faces strong opposition and is frequently dismissed as antiquarian by those who deliberately promote increasingly more complex solutions and technology in the name of "progress."

Finally, in structuring and managing programs, encourage involvement and participation of the affected population. An increasingly massive body of evidence is accumulating that suggests the positive effects of participation in organizations and programs. The manager who is sensitive to that can reap valuable dividends from the heightened sense of involvement, cooperation, and commitment that are likely to follow. In the smallpox campaign, cooperative involvement of the local population was of utmost importance. "Often the success or failure of an operation depended on the cooperation of village leaders." Studying the people's perception in order to overcome the notion that smallpox was a "disease of shame" was extremely important in many areas.[13] During the global campaign, each national program was encouraged to use its own initiative to develop appropriate local plans and approaches, even though WHO exercised a central coordination and leadership role.

Effects of the Smallpox Eradication Campaign

Any endeavor of the magnitude of the global smallpox eradication campaign inevitably produces widespread effects, often far beyond the immediate problem area of the effort. This was surely true in the case of smallpox, although in retrospect we are likely to fail to appreciate the staggering achievements of the campaign. This lack of appreciation is evident not only in the more developed countries (most of which eliminated smallpox many years ago) but also in some of recently endemic countries of the world (mostly the less developed nations). Sadly enough, in many of the latter, smallpox had been relegated for so long as a disease of the lower classes that many people—those not affected directly—scarcely noted its disappearance.

Despite these reservations, the effects of the campaign are profound. As Lawrence Altman, a participant, later observed, the campaign

> boosted interest in the global aspects of medicine by pointing up how relatively simple measures could help suppress many infections in the third world that the developed countries controlled long ago.
>
> [It] stimulated many researchers who had confined themselves to the ivory tower approach toward tropical diseases to become interested in applying their skills to seek better treatments of the diseases that are everyday problems in the developing countries.[14]

It is probably true that the unquestioned success of the smallpox campaign contributed to the beginning of an attitudinal change in WHO and perhaps to the creation of a new enthusiasm in that organization. Some of the principal participants in the global campaign detect the development of new boldness in WHO and stronger credibility for the organization. WHO's attacks in the Expanded Program of Immunization, the diarrhea program, the special tropical disease and leprosy programs, all employ forms of vertical organization and more important, evince the belief in WHO that concentrated attacks can control or eradicate other disease plagues. These examples do not indicate at all that a thoroughgoing reversal of dominant WHO thinking has occurred. The majority of WHO personnel probably still favor horizontal, integrated programs of health care. But, at least, "the success of the smallpox eradication program emphasizes the appropriateness of a single disease approach in some situations."[15] One senior official saw nothing wrong with vertical programs such as the smallpox eradication program when appropriate, but all factors must be right. There must be concern for maintenance problems after the vertical programs.[16]

A great value in vertical programs is their effect in "establishing the cutting edge" and laying foundations for other programs. Even where the smallpox eradication campaign failed to leave something behind it, the campaign was still worth the cost and effort. And people who are negative in that respect may be underestimating the residual effects. For example, "surveillance" is now a common word in health. The smallpox campaign said, in effect, look at a global problem and decide how to assemble resources and work together.[17]

Undoubtedly one of the most important effects of the smallpox campaign was the precedent it established. It clearly demonstrated the feasibility of international cooperation on a large scale. It proved "that a communicable disease can be eradicated globally" and in that respect it breached "an important psychological barrier." In many respects, the campaign boosted the confidence of epidemiologists that they could combine technological advances in disease control with natural epidemiologic factors so as to raise effectiveness. (This was the underlying rationale of the Nigerian experience that led to the surveillance-containment strategy.) The campaign also provided a massive test of various epidemiologic approaches on a scale never before attempted, and it proved the practicality and efficacy of those approaches.[18]

General Observations and Conclusions

As much as anything, the smallpox eradication campaign demonstrated what the proper application of great organizational talent and energy can accomplish. But such talent and energy must be combined with an appropriate objective and sufficient resources.

In the case of smallpox, various elements combined in such a way as to make the eradication of the disease feasible. Smallpox was the right disease to attack—my impression is that virtually all the participants in the campaign recognize that. This is no way diminishes the achievement, but it should make us cautious in regard to the transferability of the lessons learned from the experience.

It should be recognized also that most of the accomplishments of the smallpox eradication campaign (surveillance-containment, the bifurcated needle, freeze-dried vaccine, etc.) were not so much really innovations as they were the product of the long fermentation of ideas, slowly accumulating experience, and years of development.[19] This observation suggests the vital importance of information retrieval, collation, and interpretation as prime management tools. As Donald Hopkins notes,

> The smallpox eradication program is a reminder of the unfortunate delay between discovery and implementation of key medical advances. The history of smallpox eradication reveals repeated instances of critical knowledge which lay unapplied for decades.[20]

Hopkins goes on to record examples of such delay. Even when Jenner published his *Inquiry into the Causes and Effects of the Variola Vaccinae* (1798), laypersons had been inoculating cowpox material to prevent smallpox for over 24 years. The use of glycerine to preserve vaccine lymph was advocated in print in 1850 and 1869, but was not widely used until Copeman's published account of glycerine's germicidal effect in 1891. France and the Netherlands used dried smallpox vaccine in their colonies beginning in the 1920's, but preservation by freeze-drying was largely ignored until the smallpox outbreak in New York City in 1947. (The many references in epidemiologic literature to the surveillance-containment approach—long before the Nigerian experience of 1967–1968—have been noted above.)

Undoubtedly, many other examples of "lost" knowledge and delays between discovery and implementation could be noted. In part, all this suggests the importance of *appropriate timing* in administration as well as in technology. In many respects, the timing was *right* for the second global smallpox eradication campaign. It is quite arguable that not until 1966 were the World Health Assembly, WHO, and the international community *ready* to undertake an effort of such magnitude.

If we press that argument too far, however, it becomes an argument for fatalism. In truth, much of the course of developments in technology, epidemiologic knowledge, and even political will is amenable to human intervention. Regrettably, much of the blame for delay, for failure to exploit existing technology, for neglect in application of knowledge, must be placed squarely upon fallible humans.

That is precisely why the smallpox eradication campaign can serve to illuminate our way in future efforts to control or eradicate diseases. No more than that should be claimed, although the campaign represents human effort at its best.

The success of the smallpox campaign should serve also to encourage a careful examination of the desirability and efficacy of broad, comprehensive health programs. Generally this remains the approach favored by WHO, and although the goal of "good health for all" is laudable, there are serious dangers connected with it. As Holger Lundbeck has cautioned, there is the risk that "the butter will be spread so thin over the bread that you will not be able to feel the taste of it."[21] There is the ever-present danger that excessively ambitious comprehensive health programs will degenerate into rhetoric and inaction. Nothing clears the head like intimidating statistics on the number of smallpox cases in Bihar state, for example. But vague objectives such as "assuring access of all to primary health care facilities" are as likely to conceal lethargy as they are to insure health care. There is serious doubt that sufficient trained people, health care, infrastructure, and funds exist (or would be allocated) for such a sweeping program. As an alternative, Walsh and Warren have proposed an approach called "selective primary health care." This approach would focus on "preventing or treating the few diseases that are responsible for the greatest mortality and morbidity and. . .for which interventions of proved efficacy exist." The diseases that should receive highest priority include diarrheal disease, measles, malaria, whooping cough, and neonatal tetanus, and in some countries, schistosomiasis.[22] Program managers should be held strictly accountable for the accomplishment of precise, clear, measurable goals. Nothing less is likely to lead the world to higher levels of health for all people.

WHO, and the world's health care systems, can learn much from the overall legacy of the smallpox eradication campaign. As Nicole Grasset remembered,

> What we have left behind . . . is a way of tackling a problem, not just a disease. . . . Our way of thinking was "What is going wrong?" "Why?" "What must be done?" . . . "How shall we implement the new plan of action?" and then "How shall we assess its success?"[23]

The smallpox campaign offers also a commentary on relations between less developed countries and developed countries and on the capability of less developed countries for self-help in disease control and other areas. Overall, the amount of outside aid in the campaign was quite small. To this extent, the campaign demonstrated that many less developed countries can achieve important social goals without major outside assistance. Whether the residual effects of the campaign led to any substantial modification or improvement in the health systems of the countries involved is indeterminate. (Several participants believe that, in many countries, the lessons of the campaign were lost because of obdurate bureaucracies and traditional ways.)

From another perspective, there can be little doubt that the smallpox eradication campaign, focused primarily at endemic countries of the less developed world, benefitted the populations of industrialized, more developed ones enormously. Analyzed from this perspective in terms of costs and benefits, the smallpox eradication campaign was one of the greatest bargains in the history of international assistance.

Postscript

It is said that at a meeting in Kenya in 1978 the director-general of WHO, on announcing the end of smallpox, turned to D. A. Henderson and asked which was the next disease to be eradicated. Henderson reached for the microphone and said that the next disease that needs to be eradicated is bad management.[24]

Perhaps that is the moral of this story.

Notes

1. I. Arita, "Virological evidence for the success of the smallpox eradication programme," 279 *Nature* (24 May 1979), 293.
2. Nicole Grasset, "Faith and Determination," *World Health* (August-September 1976), 38–39.
3. Interview, J. Donald Millar (CDC), 15 May 1981.
4. Letter, Holger Lundbeck to I. Arita (WHO), 7 February 1980.
5. Interview, Ralph H. Henderson (WHO), 6 October 1981.
6. Chris Argyris, "Making the Undiscussable and Its Undiscussability Discussable," 40 *Public Administration Review* (May/June 1980), 206.
7. E. A. Morinis, "Two Pathways in Understanding Disease: Traditional and Scientific," 32 *WHO Chronicle* (1978), 59.
8. S. O. Foster, "Smallpox eradication: lessons learned in Bangladesh." 31 *WHO Chronicle* (1977), 245–247.
9. D. A. Henderson, "Epidemiology in the Global Eradication of Smallpox." 1 *International Journal of Epidemiology* (Spring 1972), 28.
10. Interview, Walter Orenstein (CDC), 8 May 1981.
11. Interview, J. Donald Millar (CDC), 15 May 1981.
12. Donald R. Hopkins letter dated 9 January 1980 to I. Arita, WHO.

13. Stanley Foster, "Smallpox Eradication: Lessons learned in Bangladesh," 31 *WHO Chronicle* (1977), 245–247.

14. Lawrence K. Altman, "The Doctor's World: The Eradication of Smallpox," *The New York Times,* 16 October 1979, p. C3.

15. Letter, Donald R. Hopkins (CDC) to I. Arita (WHO), 9 January 1980.

16. Interview, I. D. Ladnyi (WHO), 20 November 1981.

17. Interview, William H. Foege (CDC), 14 May 1981.

18. Letter, Donald R. Hopkins (CDC) to I. Arita (WHO), 9 January 1980.

19. This observation might apply even to the premier role usually attributed to Edward Jenner in the development of smallpox vaccine. Peter Razzell suggests the controversial thesis that "the vaccine used by Edward Jenner, after his initial trial experiments with cowpox inoculation, were derived not from cowpox but from smallpox, and that the bulk of the vaccine used for the first forty years or so of the nineteenth century was an attenuated strain of smallpox virus." What Razzell concludes is that Jenner's contribution was only part of "a long history of smallpox prophylaxis, which includes both variolation and vaccination, stretching over hundreds, and perhaps even thousands of years." Peter Razzel, *Edward Jenner's Cowpox Vaccine: The History of a Medical Myth* (Sussex: Caliban Press, 1977), pp. 5 and 107.

20. Letter, Donald R. Hopkins (CDC) to I. Arita (WHO), 9 January 1980.

21. Letter, Holger Lundbeck to I. Arita (WHO), 7 February 1980.

22. Julia A. Walsh and Kenneth S. Warren, "Selective Primary Health Care: An Interim Strategy for Disease Control in Developing Countries," 301 *New England Journal of Medicine* (1979), 967–974, cited in Avis Berman, "Health Care in the Poorer World: An Interim Strategy," 5 *RF Illustrated* (October 1980), 10.

23. N. Grasset, "Faith and Determination," *World Health* (August-September, 1976), 39.

24. Interview, R. C. Hogan (WHO), 2 December 1981.

Index

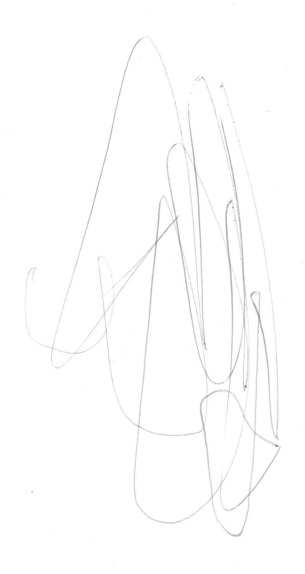

0680

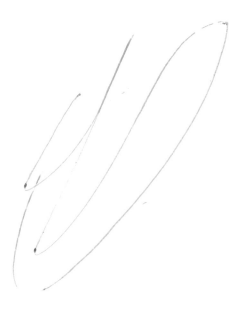